Complete OSCE Skills for Medical and Surgical Finals

Complete OSCE Skills for Medical and Surgical Finals

KATE TATHAM BSc (HONS) MB BS MRCP FRCA
Specialty Registrar, Anaesthetics and Intensive Care Medicine
Imperial School of Anaesthesia
London, UK

KINESH PATEL BA (HONS) MB BS MRCP
Specialty Registrar, Gastroenterology
Chelsea and Westminster NHS Foundation Trust
London, UK

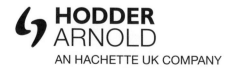

**HODDER
ARNOLD**

AN HACHETTE UK COMPANY

First published in Great Britain in 2010 by
Hodder Arnold, an imprint of Hodder Education, an Hachette UK company,
338 Euston Road, London NW1 3BH

http://www.hoddereducation.com

British Library Cataloguing in Publication Data
A catalogue record for this book is available from the British Library

Library of Congress Cataloging-in-Publication Data
A catalog record for this book is available from the Library of Congress

ISBN 978-0-340-97424-7

1 2 3 4 5 6 7 8 9 10

Commissioning Editor: Joanna Koster
Project Editor: Sarah Penny
Production Controller: Karen Dyer and Kate Harris
Cover Design: Amina Dudhia

Typeset in 10 on 13pt Minion by Phoenix Photosetting, Chatham, Kent
Printed and bound in India

What do you think about this book? Or any other Hodder Arnold title?
Please visit our website: www.hoddereducation.com

Contents

To our partners and families

Preface

Clinical examinations are a stressful but necessary part of medical school finals. However, with the appropriate preparation and practice they can become significantly less daunting and even an opportunity to prove your clinical skills.

The aim of this book is to help in this process of revision by providing an overview of common clinical situations encountered in OSCE stations. This quick reference text allows you and your peers to test each other's skills both at the bedside and in role play scenarios.

Although this book has not been written as an exhaustive guide, it provides the essential knowledge necessary to succeed in your exams.

Good luck!

Acknowledgements

We would like to thank **Dr Andrew Thillainayagam** for his help and guidance.

We would also like to thank the following for their contributions and advice:

- **Heidi Artis BSc, MB BS**
  Specialty Registrar
  Acute Care Common Stem, Anaesthetics & Intensive Care

- **Catherine Bennett BSc, MB BS, DFSRH**
  General Practice Registrar

- **Sarita Depani BSc, MB BS, MRCPCH**
  Specialty Registrar
  Paediatrics

- **Rebecca Evans-Jones BA, MB BS, MRCOG**
  Specialty Registrar
  Obstetrics and Gynaecology

- **Lucy Hicks BSc, MB BS, MRCP**
  Specialty Registrar
  Gastroenterology

- **James Waller BSc, MB BS, MRCP**
  Specialty Registrar
  Cardiology

We would especially like to thank **Paolo Sorelli** for his continuing support, helpful comments and enthusiasm.

List of abbreviations

5-HT	5-hydroxytryptamine
AAA	abdominal aortic aneurysm
ACE	angiotensin-converting enzyme
ACTH	adrenocorticotropic hormone
AF	atrial fibrillation
AFP	α-fetoprotein
AIDS	acquired immune deficiency syndrome
AP	anteroposterior
ASIS	anterior superior iliac spine
BCC	basal cell carcinoma
BMI	body mass index
CABG	coronary artery bypass graft
CAPD	continuous ambulatory peritoneal dialysis
CIN	cervical intraepithelial neoplasia
CK	creatine kinase
CNS	central nervous system
COPD	chronic obstructive pulmonary disease
COX-2	cyclo-oxygenase-2
CPR	cardiopulmonary resuscitation
CRP	C-reactive protein
CSF	cerebrospinal fluid
CT	computed tomography
CTG	cardiotocograph
CXR	chest radiograph
DIP	distal interphalangeal
DMARD	disease modifying antirheumatic drug
DNR	do not resuscitate
ECG	electrocardiogram
EEG	electroencephalography
EMG	electromyography
ESR	erythrocyte sedimentation rate
FBC	full blood count
FEV_1	forced expiratory volume in 1 second
FiO_2	fraction of inspired oxygen

FSH	follicle stimulating hormone
FVC	forced vital capacity
GCA	giant cell arteritis
GCS	Glasgow Coma Scale
GP	general practitioner
GTN	glyceryl trinitrate
HIV	human immunodeficiency virus
HLA	human leucocyte antigen
HOCM	hypertrophic obstructive cardiomyopathy
HRT	hormone replacement therapy
HSMN	hereditary sensory and motor neuropathy
ICE	ideas, concerns and expectations
ICP	intracranial pressure
IPF	idiopathic pulmonary fibrosis
IUGR	intrauterine growth restriction
JVP	jugular venous pressure
LDH	lactate dehydrogenase
LFT	liver function tests
LH	luteinizing hormone
LMN	lower motor neurone
LMP	last menstrual period
LUQ	left upper quadrant
MCP	metacarpophalangeal
MDI	metered-dose inhaler
MI	myocardial infarction
MMR	measles, mumps and rubella
NSAID	non-steroidal anti-inflammatory drug
OSA	obstructive sleep apnoea
PALS	Patient Advice and Liaison Service
PCI	percutaneous coronary intervention
PCKD	polycystic kidney disease
PEFR	peak expiratory flow rate
PEP	post-exposure prophylaxis
PET	positron emission tomography
PFT	pulmonary function test
PID	pelvic inflammatory disease
PIP	proximal interphalangeal
PND	paroxysmal nocturnal dyspnoea
POC	products of conception
PUO	pyrexia of unknown origin
RIF	right iliac fossa
RUQ	right upper quadrant
SACD	subacute combined degeneration of the cord
SCC	squamous cell carcinoma
SFH	symphysis–fundal height
SFJ	saphenofemoral junction

STI	sexually transmitted infection
SVT	supraventricular tachycardia
TIA	transient ischaemic attack
U&E	urea and electrolytes
UMN	upper motor neurone
UTI	urinary tract infection
VT	ventricular tachycardia

History

HISTORY TAKING SKILLS

Familiarity with the key components of a history is invaluable when taking a history from any patient.

INTRODUCTION
- Introduce yourself to the patient
- Confirm the reason for the interview
- Ensure the patient is sitting comfortably, alongside and not behind a desk

PATIENT DETAILS
- Confirm the patient's details:
  - Full name
  - Age and date of birth
  - Occupation

PRESENTING COMPLAINT
- Ask the patient to describe their problem by using open questions
- The presenting complaint should be expressed in their own words, e.g. 'heaviness in the chest'
- Do not interrupt their first few sentences
- Try to elicit their ideas, concerns and expectations (ICE)

HISTORY OF PRESENTING COMPLAINT
- Interrogate the patient further about the presenting complaint
- A useful guide, e.g. for pain, is the mnemonic 'SOCRATES'
  - **S**ite
  - **O**nset
  - **C**haracter

- ○ **R**adiation
- ○ **A**lleviating factors
- ○ **T**iming
- ○ **E**xacerbating factors
- ○ **S**everity scale (1–10)
- ○ And associated **S**ymptoms

PAST MEDICAL HISTORY

- Enquire about diseases relating to the presenting complaint. For example, for chest pain:
  - ○ Coronary heart disease/angina/myocardial infarction
  - ○ Indigestion/reflux/hiatus hernia
  - ○ Asthma/chronic obstructive pulmonary disease (COPD)/pulmonary fibrosis
  - ○ Deep vein thrombosis/pulmonary embolism/hypercoagulability
- Ask all patients if they have a history of important diseases (mnemonic 'MJ THREADS Ca'):
  - ○ Myocardial infarction
  - ○ Jaundice
  - ○ Tuberculosis
  - ○ Hypertension
  - ○ Rheumatic fever
  - ○ Epilepsy
  - ○ Asthma
  - ○ Diabetes
  - ○ Stroke
  - ○ Cancer

DRUG HISTORY

- Enquire about all medications including creams, drops, the oral contraceptive and herbal/vitamin preparations
- Specify:
  - ○ Route
  - ○ Dose
  - ○ Frequency
  - ○ Compliance
- Take a detailed allergy history, e.g. which medications/foods and the symptoms

FAMILY HISTORY

- Ask the patient about any relevant family diseases, e.g. coronary heart disease, diabetes
- Enquire about the patient's parents, and the cause of death if deceased
- Sketch a short family tree, including any offspring (Fig. 1.1)

SOCIAL (AND PSYCHIATRIC) HISTORY

- Assess any alcohol use in approximate units/week
- Ask about tobacco use – quantify with 'pack years' (number of packets of 20 cigarettes smoked per day multiplied by number of years smoking)
- Employment history, including exposure to pathogens, e.g. asbestos

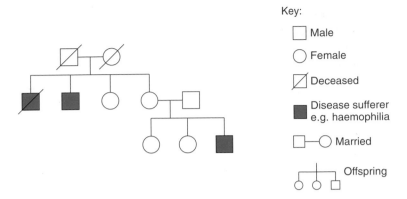

Key:

□ Male

○ Female

⊘ Deceased

■ Disease sufferer
e.g. haemophilia

□—○ Married

Offspring

Figure 1.1 Example family tree

- Enquire about home situation, including any pets
- Enquire about any history of psychiatric disease

SYSTEMS REVIEW

- Run through a comprehensive list of symptoms from all systems:
  - Cardiovascular, e.g. chest pain, palpitations
  - Respiratory, e.g. cough, dyspnoea
  - Gastrointestinal, e.g. abdominal pain, diarrhoea
  - Genitourinary, e.g. dysuria, discharge
  - Neurological, e.g. numbness, weakness
  - Musculoskeletal, e.g. aches, pains
  - Psychiatric, e.g. depression, anxiety

SUMMARY

- Provide a short summary of the history including:
  - Name and age of patient
  - Presenting complaint
  - Relevant medical history
- Give a differential diagnosis (e.g. 'This could be a myocardial infarction or oesophageal spasm')
- Formulate a short investigation and treatment plan

CHEST PAIN

INTRODUCTION

- Introduce yourself
- Confirm patient's name
- Confirm reason for meeting
- Adopt appropriate body language

HISTORY OF PRESENTING COMPLAINT

The mnemonic 'SOCRATES' is useful for assessing chest pain (see p. 1). Enquire about:

- **S**ite – central or left chest, retrosternal, epigastric
- **O**nset – sudden, gradual, related to trauma/exertion
- **C**haracter – crushing, heavy, tight band, pleuritic, burning
- **R**adiation – radiating to left arm, neck, jaw or back
- **A**lleviation – rest, glyceryl trinitrate (GTN) spray, sitting forward (pericarditis)
- **T**iming – related to exertion
- **E**xacerbating factors – effort, emotion, movement, food, respiration, cold weather
- **S**everity scale – 1–10
- And associated **S**ymptoms:
    - Dyspnoea, palpitations
    - Syncope/collapse
    - Sweating, burping, nausea/vomiting
    - Ankle swelling
    - Calf swelling
    - Paroxysmal nocturnal dyspnoea (PND) or orthopnoea
    - Cough, haemoptysis, sputum
    - Fever, constitutional upset, coryza
    - Panic attacks, anxiety

PAST MEDICAL HISTORY

- Vascular disease:
    - Angina, previous myocardial infarction (MI), previous angioplasty or coronary artery bypass graft (CABG) surgery
    - Claudication
    - Cerebrovascular disease, transient ischaemic attacks
    - Risk factors
        - Hypertension
        - Hyperlipidaemia
        - Diabetes
        - Smoking
        - Family history (MI <60 years, hyperlipidaemia)
- Thromboembolic disease:
    - Recent surgery, cancer, immobility
    - Inherited hypercoagulable state, e.g. protein S or C deficiency
    - Oral contraceptive/hormone replacement therapy
    - Smoking
- Pneumothorax:
    - Tall, thin man
    - Connective tissue disease (e.g. Marfan's)

DRUG HISTORY

- Cardiac medications: β-blockers, diuretics, antiplatelet agents, GTN spray
- Recreational drug use, e.g. cocaine (coronary artery spasm)
- Chronic non-steroidal anti-inflammatory drug (NSAID) use causing gastritis/oesophagitis/reflux

SOCIAL HISTORY

- Smoking
- Alcohol intake
- Diet (fatty food, salt intake)
- Lifestyle, exercise
- Recent immobility/major surgery/long-haul travel

BOX 1.1 DIFFERENTIAL DIAGNOSIS: CHEST PAIN

Cardiovascular:
- Myocardial infarction
- Acute coronary syndrome (non-ST elevation MI, unstable angina)
- Angina (induced by effort and relieved by rest)
- Acute aortic dissection
- Pericarditis

Gastrointestinal:
- Reflux oesophagitis
- Oesophageal spasm
- Peptic ulcer disease

Respiratory:
- Pulmonary embolism
- Pneumonia
- Pneumothorax

Musculoskeletal:
- Costochondritis (Tietze's syndrome)
- Chest wall injuries

Psychosomatic:
- Anxiety/depression

SHORTNESS OF BREATH

INTRODUCTION

- Introduce yourself
- Confirm patient's name
- Confirm reason for meeting
- Adopt appropriate body language

HISTORY OF PRESENTING COMPLAINT

Enquire about:

- Onset and duration – acute, chronic, constant, intermittent
- Exacerbating factors – effort, emotion, movement, cold weather
- Alleviation – rest, inhalers
- Timing – related to exertion
- Associated symptoms:
    - Wheeze
    - Stridor
    - Cough – productive or dry, colour of sputum
    - Fever, night sweats or weight loss
    - Haemoptysis – how much: teaspoon, cup-full
    - Chest pain – pleuritic, cardiac

- Palpitations
- Nausea and vomiting, sweating, dizziness
- Ankle swelling
- Paroxysmal nocturnal dyspnoea (PND)
- Orthopnoea – number of pillows
- Exercise tolerance – quantify, e.g. number of stairs, distance on the flat

PAST MEDICAL HISTORY

- Asthma: frequency of attacks, admissions to hospital or intensive care unit
- COPD: frequency of exacerbations, admissions (as for asthma), use of home oxygen (number of hours) and home nebulizers
- Recurrent lower respiratory tract infections
- Cardiac failure or structural disease
- Arrhythmias
- Deep vein thrombosis, procoagulant states (e.g. pregnancy, cancer, surgery)

DRUG HISTORY

- Nebulizers
- Cardiac medications
- Diuretics, e.g. furosemide
- Angiotensin-converting enzyme (ACE) inhibitors

FAMILY HISTORY

- History of atopy – asthma, eczema, hay fever
- Tuberculosis

SOCIAL HISTORY

- Smoking history (active and passive)
- Occupation and exposure to coal, dust, asbestos
- Animal exposure (pets, farming)
- Tuberculosis exposure
- Limitation of daily activities by shortness of breath

BOX 1.2 DIFFERENTIAL DIAGNOSIS

Acute:
- Asthma
- Acute exacerbation COPD
- Lower respiratory tract infection
- Pulmonary oedema
- Pulmonary embolism
- Pneumothorax
- Pleural effusion
- Lung cancer
- Anxiety/panic attack
- Metabolic acidosis

Chronic:
- COPD
- Cardiac failure
- Pulmonary fibrosis
- Anaemia
- Arrhythmias
- Cystic fibrosis
- Pulmonary hypertension

FEVER/PYREXIA OF UNKNOWN ORIGIN

INTRODUCTION

- Introduce yourself
- Confirm patient's name
- Confirm reason for meeting
- Adopt appropriate body language

HISTORY OF PRESENTING COMPLAINT

- Onset – sudden, gradual
- Character – constant, intermittent
- Frequency of peaks in temperature
  - Has the temperature been recorded?
- Alleviation – rest, paracetamol
- Timing – related to exertion
- Exacerbating factors – climate/weather, time of day
- Associated symptoms/signs:
  - Rigors or shivering
  - Sweating (especially at night)
  - Weight loss
  - Anorexia
  - Feeling faint or dizziness, syncopal episodes
  - Fatigue
  - Lumps, tender lymph nodes
  - Pain
  - Cough and sputum (lower respiratory tract infection)
  - Diarrhoea and vomiting, abdominal pain (gastroenteritis)
  - Urinary frequency, dysuria, haematuria (urinary tract infection [UTI])
  - Rashes or skin changes, areas of erythema (viral illnesses, cellulitis)
  - Headache, neck stiffness, photophobia (meningitis)
  - Heart failure, track marks, lethargy, rash, new murmur (infective endocarditis)

PAST MEDICAL HISTORY

- Recent surgery
- Recent illness, e.g. upper respiratory tract infection
- Blood transfusions

DRUG HISTORY

- Intravenous drug use
- Appropriate malaria prophylaxis when travelling and compliance
- Immunizations up to date

FAMILY HISTORY

- Any family members with contagious disease
- Animal – contact, bites

SEXUAL HISTORY

- Sexual history – recent sexual practice (see p. 289)

TRAVEL HISTORY

- Travel history – location, appropriate vaccinations, diet, food hygiene, swimming

SOCIAL HISTORY

- Tattoos
- Piercings
- Occupational exposure, e.g. to animals

BOX 1.3 COMMON DIFFERENTIAL DIAGNOSES OF PYREXIA OF UNKNOWN ORIGIN

Infective:
- Bacterial: e.g. pneumonia, urinary tract infection, meningitis, endocarditis, abdominal/pelvic abscess
- Viral: e.g. gastroenteritis, hepatitis, HIV seroconversion
- Parasitic: e.g. malaria, schistosomiasis

Inflammatory: e.g. systemic lupus erythematosus, rheumatoid arthritis, Crohn's disease

Malignancy: e.g. lymphoma, leukaemia, hepatocellular carcinoma

Others: e.g. pulmonary embolus, factitious, recent vaccination, thyrotoxicosis

---

INVESTIGATIONS

There are numerous investigations, depending on the history, including:

- FBC, urea and electrolytes (U&E), liver function tests (LFTs), C-reactive protein (CRP), erythrocyte sedimentation rate (ESR), viral screen, Toxoplasma antibodies, Paul Bunnell test, thyroid function tests
- Hepatitis screen
- Blood cultures
- Sputum culture
- Mid-stream urinalysis
- Stool culture
- CXR
- ECG

For difficult cases, echocardiography (endocarditis), CT and positron emission tomography (PET) can help localize abnormalities giving rise to the fever.

ABDOMINAL PAIN

INTRODUCTION

- Introduce yourself
- Confirm patient's name
- Confirm reason for meeting
- Adopt appropriate body language

HISTORY OF PRESENTING COMPLAINT

Enquire about:

- **S**ite – where did it start and has it moved?
- **O**nset – sudden, gradual
- **C**haracter – crampy, colicky, sharp, burning
- **R**adiation – e.g. loin to groin (renal colic)
- **A**lleviation – relieved by opening bowels or vomiting?
- **T**iming – related to eating/bowels/micturition/menstruation/movement?
- **E**xacerbating factors
- **S**everity scale – 1–10, does it wake you?
- Associated **S**ymptoms:
  - Nausea and vomiting – haematemesis, coffee-grounds, bile-stained or feculent?
  - Dysphagia
  - Dyspepsia
  - Change in bowel habit – diarrhoea/constipation, altered frequency, colour, consistency, pale, offensive smell, frothy, hard to flush away (steatorrhoea), blood or mucus present
  - Rectal bleeding
  - Bloating, flatulence
  - Weight gain/loss
  - Appetite change
  - Jaundice, pruritus, dark urine, pale stools
  - Rigors/fever
  - Haematuria, dysuria, vaginal discharge

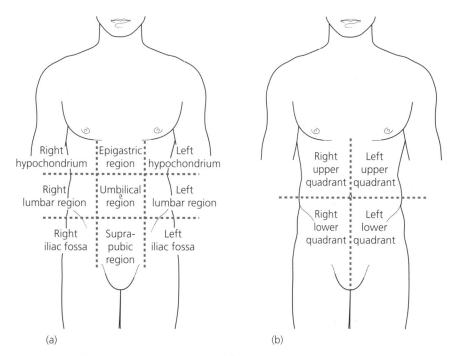

(a)   (b)

Figure 1.2 Areas of the abdomen: (a) ninths or (b) quadrants

PAST MEDICAL HISTORY

- Inflammatory bowel disease – Crohn's, ulcerative colitis
- Diverticular disease
- Previous abdominal/pelvic surgery (adhesions causing bowel obstruction)
- Recent trauma or injury (e.g. splenic rupture)
- Menstruation (pregnant/ectopic) and sexual history (pelvic inflammatory disease)
- Other common diseases: MJ THREADS Ca (see p. 2)

DRUG HISTORY

- NSAIDs
- Laxatives
- Opiates
- Antibiotics, e.g. erythromycin

FAMILY HISTORY

- Inflammatory bowel disease
- Polyps, bowel cancer
- Jaundice
- Family members with diarrhoea and vomiting

SOCIAL HISTORY

- Alcohol intake
- Recreational drug use
- Travel abroad
- Recent potentially infected food intake
- Blood transfusions, tattoos
- Sexual history (see p. 289)

BOX 1.4 DIFFERENTIAL DIAGNOSIS OF ABDOMINAL PAIN

Gastrointestinal:
- Gastritis, dyspepsia, peptic ulcer disease (PUD)
- Appendicitis
- Peritonitis
- Perforated gastric ulcer
- Bowel obstruction
- Diverticulitis
- Gastroenteritis
- Inflammatory bowel disease
- Mesenteric adenitis
- Strangulated hernia
- Volvulus
- Intussusception
- Irritable bowel syndrome
- Pancreatitis
- Malignancy

Hepatobiliary:
- Cholangitis
- Acute cholecystitis
- Cholelithiasis (gall stones)
- Hepatitis
- Fitz–Hugh–Curtis syndrome (chlamydial perihepatitis)

Splenic:
- Infarction
- Rupture

Genitourinary:
- Acute pyelonephritis
- Renal colic
- Cystitis/urinary tract infection
- Ectopic pregnancy
- Torsion or rupture of ovarian cyst
- Pelvic inflammatory disease
- Salpingitis
- Endometriosis
- Fibroids
- Dysmenorrhoea
- Referred pain of testicular torsion

Other:
- Abdominal aortic aneurysm
- Mesenteric thrombosis or embolus
- Diabetic ketoacidosis
- Sickle cell crisis
- Acute porphyria
- Acute MI

CHANGE IN BOWEL HABIT

INTRODUCTION

- Introduce yourself
- Confirm patient's name
- Confirm reason for meeting
- Adopt appropriate body language

HISTORY OF PRESENTING COMPLAINT

Enquire about:

- Normal bowel habit (for patient)
- Changes:
  - Symptoms:
    - Frequency of bowel opening
    - Constipation
    - Diarrhoea – watery, loose

- Steatorrhoea – pale, offensive smell, frothy, hard to flush away
- Rectal blood – mixed in, on paper, in toilet pan, altered or frank blood
- Any pus, slime or mucus
  - Onset – sudden, gradual
  - Duration
  - Timing – any relation to food, menstruation, activity level, time of day
  - Alleviating factors – e.g. certain food avoidance
  - Exacerbating factors – e.g. exercise, sleep patterns, food
  - Associated symptoms:
    - Nausea and vomiting – haematemesis, coffee-grounds, bile-stained or feculent
    - Dysphagia
    - Dyspepsia
    - Bloating, flatulence
    - Weight gain/loss
    - Appetite change, diet change
    - Jaundice, pruritus, dark urine, pale stools
    - Rigors/fever
    - Haematuria, dysuria, vaginal discharge

PAST MEDICAL HISTORY

- Inflammatory bowel disease – Crohn's, ulcerative colitis
- Coeliac disease
- Diverticular disease
- Groin/midline/incisional hernias
- Previous abdominal surgery (e.g. adhesions causing bowel obstruction)
- Metabolic disturbances, e.g. thyroid disease

DRUG HISTORY

- NSAIDs
- Laxatives
- Opiates
- Antibiotics, e.g. erythromycin

FAMILY HISTORY

- Inflammatory bowel disease
- Polyps, bowel cancer
- Family members with diarrhoea and vomiting

SOCIAL HISTORY

- Alcohol intake
- Recreational drug use
- Travel abroad
- Recent potentially infected food intake
- Sexual history (see p. 289)

BOX 1.5 DIFFERENTIAL DIAGNOSIS OF CHANGE IN BOWEL HABIT

Gastrointestinal:
- Appendicitis
- Peritonitis
- Perforated gastric ulcer
- Bowel obstruction
- Ileus, e.g. postoperative
- Diverticulitis
- Gastroenteritis
- Inflammatory bowel disease (Crohn's or ulcerative colitis)
- Strangulated hernia
- Volvulus
- Intussusception
- Irritable bowel syndrome
- Pancreatitis
- Malignancy
- Biliary obstruction, e.g. gallstones
- Anal pain, e.g. fissure, fistula

Infective:
- Bacterial, e.g. *Salmonella* species
- Viral
- Fungal
- Protozoan

Drugs:
- Opiates
- Laxatives
- Antibiotics
- Tricyclic antidepressants

Metabolic:
- Thyroid disease
- Diabetes (autonomic disease)
- Carcinoid

Others:
- Anxiety
- Depression
- Diet

TIREDNESS

INTRODUCTION
- Introduce yourself
- Confirm patient's name
- Confirm reason for meeting
- Adopt appropriate body language

HISTORY OF PRESENTING COMPLAINT

Enquire about:

- Onset and duration:
  - Sudden onset and short history, e.g. post-viral cause
  - Long duration (more suggestive of emotional origin)
- Related factors:
  - If related to exertion – more likely organic cause
  - Time of day, e.g. rheumatoid arthritis worse on waking
  - Improved after rest, e.g. myasthenia gravis
- Associated symptoms:
  - Weight loss, anorexia, dyspnoea – suggest underlying pathology, e.g. cancer
  - Weight gain, constipation, dry skin and hair, cold intolerance – e.g. hypothyroidism
  - Chronic pain
  - Rectal bleeding, abdominal pain, menorrhagia, e.g. anaemia

- Sleep patterns:
  - ○ Early morning waking – depression
  - ○ Snoring, daytime somnolence, early morning headaches, obesity – obstructive sleep apnoea (OSA) (see Box 1.6)

BOX 1.6 EPWORTH SLEEPINESS SCALE – ESTABLISHES POSSIBLE DIAGNOSIS OF OSA

For each question score for chance of dozing (0 = no chance, 1 = slight, 2 = moderate, 3 = high; score >11/24 significant)

Likelihood of falling asleep when:
- Sitting and reading
- Watching television
- Sitting inactive in a public place
- Passenger in a car for 1 hour
- Lying down to rest in the afternoon
- Sitting and talking to someone
- Sitting quietly after lunch (without alcohol)
- Sitting in the car in traffic for few minutes

PAST MEDICAL HISTORY

- Recent viral illnesses
- Sleep apnoea
- Cardiac disease
- Hypothyroidism (or previous thyroid-related treatment including surgery)
- Endocrine diseases including diabetes mellitus
- Renal failure
- Psychiatric problems

DRUG HISTORY

- Thyroid-related medications or treatments   •
- Recent changes in dose of regular medication
- Use of analgesics and sedatives

FAMILY HISTORY

- Endocrine dysfunction

SOCIAL HISTORY

- Impact on work, family and relationships
- Occupation and exposure to chemicals or toxins
- Alcohol – i.e. excess, especially in the evenings

SYSTEMS REVIEW

Full systems review to elicit symptoms overlooked by patient.

BOX 1.7 DIFFERENTIAL DIAGNOSIS OF TIREDNESS

- Anaemia
- Hypo- or hyperthyroidism
- Malignancy
- Sleep apnoea
- Infections
- Diabetes mellitus
- Inflammatory conditions, e.g. rheumatoid arthritis

- Chronic pain
- Post-viral syndrome
- Chronic fatigue syndrome
- Fibromyalgia
- Medication side effects
- Depression, anxiety, chronic stress
- Insomnia

HEADACHE

INTRODUCTION

- Introduce yourself
- Confirm patient's name
- Confirm reason for meeting
- Adopt appropriate body language

HISTORY OF PRESENTING COMPLAINT

Enquire about:

- **S**ite
  - Where did it start, has it moved?
  - Unilateral: migraine, cluster headache, giant cell (temporal) arteritis giant cell arteritis (GCA)
  - Bilateral: tension headache, subarachnoid headache
- **O**nset – sudden, e.g. 'thunder-clap', gradual
- **C**haracter:
  - 'Tight band' or pressure – tension headache
  - Throbbing/dull ache – migraine
  - Lancinating – trigeminal neuralgia
  - Tender to touch (e.g. on combing hair) – temporal arteritis
- **R**adiation – e.g. throat, eye, ear, nose – neuralgia
- **A**lleviation – relieved by analgesia, posture, darkened room (migraine), sleep
- **T**iming and frequency:
  - Migraines 24–72 hours, cyclical in nature
  - Cluster headaches >1 hour
  - Neuralgia; paroxysms of seconds to minutes
  - Raised intracranial pressure (ICP) – worse on waking
- **E**xacerbating factors:
  - Loud noises (phonophobia), bright light (photophobia)
  - Bending/straining (with raised ICP)
  - High body mass index (BMI), steroid or oral contraceptive use – idiopathic intracranial hypertension

- **S**everity scale – 1–10, does it wake you?
- And associated **S**ymptoms:
  - ○ Aura, visual disturbances
  - ○ Nausea and vomiting
  - ○ Neck pain

BOX 1.8 INSIDIOUS FEATURES OF HEADACHE

- Sudden onset, 'thunderclap' headache
- Stiff neck
- Severe or 'worst ever' headache
- Progressively worsening headache
- Altered level of consciousness
- Progressive neurological deficit
- Recent head injury
- Meningism (photophobia, neck stiffness)
- Focal neurology
- Temporal artery tenderness
- Features suggestive of raised ICP, e.g. vomiting, posture-related headache, papilloedema

---

PAST MEDICAL HISTORY

- Depression/anxiety
- Head trauma
- Seizures
- Space-occupying lesions
- Hypertension
- Hypercoagulable states (e.g. protein S or C deficiency)

BOX 1.9 DIFFERENTIAL DIAGNOSIS OF HEADACHE

Acute:
- Subarachnoid haemorrhage
- Intracranial haemorrhage
- Meningitis
- Acute glaucoma
- Trauma
- Sinusitis
- Drugs, e.g. GTN
- Post dural puncture
- Pre-eclampsia

Chronic:
- Tension headache
- Cluster headache
- Migraine
- Analgesic rebound headache
- Tumour
- Abscess
- Venous sinus thrombosis
- Idiopathic intracranial hypertension
- Depression, anxiety

DRUG HISTORY

- Analgesia – any relief from it, recurrent use (i.e. analgesic rebound headaches)
- Serotonin (5-hydroxytryptamine [5-HT]$_3$) agonists
- Oral contraceptive use (associated with idiopathic intracranial hypertension and venous sinus thrombosis)
- Anticoagulants – high risk of intracranial bleeding if taking warfarin

SOCIAL HISTORY

- Alcohol
- Relationship and employment situation, any potential problems

COLLAPSE

INTRODUCTION

- Introduce yourself
- Confirm patient's name
- Confirm reason for meeting
- Adopt appropriate body language

HISTORY OF PRESENTING COMPLAINT

- Does the patient recall the event?
- Is there a collateral history?
- What were the exact circumstances:
  - Mechanical fall, i.e. trip or slip
  - Sport or exertion related
  - Head movement (e.g. carotid sinus syncope or vertigo/dizziness)
  - Neck extension/looking up (vertebrobasilar insufficiency)
  - On standing up (postural hypotension) or sitting down
  - Cough/micturition (syncope)
  - Emotional stress
- Prodromal symptoms:
  - Sweating, feeling faint, nausea
  - Blurred vision, aura
  - Vertigo, dizziness, tinnitus
  - Chest pain, palpitations
  - Headache or neck pain
- Did the patient lose consciousness?
  - Do they recall falling to or hitting the ground?
  - Do they recall coming round?
  - How long were they unconscious for and was this witnessed?
  - Did they feel confused or sleepy post collapse (i.e. post ictal)?
- Other symptoms:
  - Tongue biting, incontinence, any other injuries from falling
  - Headache, weakness or difficulty speaking afterwards

- Is there an eyewitness account of shaking or twitching, foaming at the mouth or being unresponsive?

PAST MEDICAL HISTORY

- Previous syncope/collapse/similar attacks
- History of arrhythmias or cardiovascular disease
- History of seizures/epilepsy/neurological diseases or surgery
- Diabetes mellitus (how well is it controlled?)
- Recent illness

FAMILY HISTORY

- Sudden cardiac death/cardiomyopathy
- Arrhythmias
- Diabetes

DRUG HISTORY

- Insulin, antidiabetic medications
- Antihypertensives (diuretics)
- Nitrates
- Sedatives
- Recent dose changes or concurrent illnesses
- Illicit drug use

SOCIAL HISTORY

- Alcohol abuse
- Older patients – social situation: do they live alone, are they coping, how good is their mobility, are they at risk of falls?

BOX 1.10 DIFFERENTIAL DIAGNOSIS OF COLLAPSE

Cardiovascular:
- Arrhythmia – sick sinus syndrome, Stokes–Adams attacks, supraventricular tachycardias (SVTs), ventricular tachycardias (VTs), heart block, bradycardias
- Valvular – cardiac outflow obstruction with aortic stenosis or hypertrophic obstructive cardiomyopathy (HOCM)
- Postural hypotension – drug induced, hypovolaemic, autonomic
- Vasovagal syncope
- Myocardial infarction
- Pulmonary embolism
- Carotid sinus syndrome (hypersensitivity)

Neurological:
- Transient ischaemic attack (TIA) or stroke
- Seizures
- Intracranial lesion

Metabolic:
- Hypo- or hyperglycaemia
- Alcohol related

Other:
- Hypoxia or hyperventilation
- Anxiety/panic attack
- Situation syncope – cough/micturition, emotional 'faints'

ALCOHOL MISUSE

INTRODUCTION

- Introduce yourself
- Confirm patient's name
- Confirm reason for meeting
- Adopt appropriate body language

PRESENTING COMPLAINT

- Can present in a number of different ways:
  - Request from the patient for help with their drinking
  - Concerned relative or friend
  - Stress, depression, anxiety
  - Memory loss
  - Lethargy and fatigue
  - Systemic symptoms: e.g. gastritis, jaundice, liver failure, encephalopathy
- Level of alcohol consumption – try to quantify in units/week
- 'CAGE' questionnaire – see Box 1.11

BOX 1.11 CAGE QUESTIONNAIRE

2 or more 'yes' = excessive drinking
- **C –** Have you ever felt you should **C**ut down on your drinking?
- **A –** Have you ever felt **A**nnoyed or **A**ngry by people criticizing your drinking?
- **G –** Have you ever felt **G**uilty about your drinking?
- **E –** Do you ever need a drink first thing in the morning? (**E**ye-opener)

- Important questions to ask:
  - Any memory loss?
  - What happens if you stop?
  - Any withdrawal symptoms – hallucinations (delirium tremens) visual or tactile or seizures?
  - Have you ever tried to give up?
  - Why did you fail?

PAST MEDICAL HISTORY/REVIEW OF SYSTEMS

Signs/symptoms of chronic liver disease:

- Jaundice
- Liver failure, ascites, weight loss
- Gastritis and peptic ulcer disease
- Upper gastrointestinal or rectal bleeding
- Pancreatitis (acute or chronic)
- Cardiomyopathy
- Head injury
- Seizures/collapse

- Peripheral neuropathy
- Korsakoff's syndrome
- Wernicke's encephalopathy

DRUG HISTORY

- Illicit drugs
- Anti-misuse therapies
- Other drug addictions

FAMILY HISTORY

- Family history of alcohol misuse
- Work or live in a public house

SOCIAL HISTORY

- Smoking history (indicator of addiction)
- Occupation (access to alcohol, e.g. work in a bar, at a brewery)
- Criminal record – drink/drive offences, record (or victim) of violence
- Relationships – is it affecting them?
- Childhood exposure to addictive behaviour

BOX 1.12 TREATING ALCOHOL MISUSE

Counselling:
- General practitioner (GP), practice nurse, self-help groups, e.g. Alcoholics Anonymous

Psychological:
- Residential units provide intensive rehabilitation regimens

Medical:
- Short-term course of sedatives to aid alcohol withdrawal
- Deterrent drugs: produce unpleasant side effects when drink alcohol
- Vitamin replacement therapy

PSYCHIATRIC HISTORY AND RISK ASSESSMENT

INTRODUCTION

- Introduce yourself
- Confirm patient's name
- Confirm reason for meeting
- Adopt appropriate body language

DEMOGRAPHY

Record the patient's:

- Age
- Gender

- Occupation
- Marital status
- Ethnicity
- Religion (if applicable)

PRESENTING COMPLAINT

Confirm the reason for referral and record in the patient's own words.

HISTORY OF PRESENTING COMPLAINT

Enquire about:

- Circumstances around presentation:
  - Stressors
  - Significant events
  - How they have affected the patient
- Any effect on/change in:
  - Sleep patterns, e.g. insomnia, early morning waking
  - Appetite, weight
  - Libido
  - Interest and enjoyment of life, e.g. anhedonia
  - Ability to concentrate
  - Memory
  - Personality, e.g. miserable, angry
  - Relationships, e.g. a break-up

PAST MEDICAL HISTORY

- Head injury
- Encephalitis, intracranial diseases
- Epilepsy
- Dementia
- Metabolic disturbance, e.g. hypothyroidism

DRUG HISTORY

- Antidepressants
- Antipsychotic agents
- Lithium – ensure therapeutic and not toxic dose
- Illicit drugs – e.g. cannabis, cocaine, heroin
- Thyroxine/antithyroid medications
- Opiates, benzodiazepines, hypnotics

PSYCHIATRIC HISTORY

- Psychiatric disease – e.g. depression, bipolar disorder
- Admissions to psychiatric institutions (voluntary/involuntary)
- Follow-up with psychiatric teams/crisis/outreach
- Treatments employed – successful?

FAMILY HISTORY

- Sketch a basic family tree including:
  - Ages
  - Health – especially mental health problems
  - History of learning disability, epilepsy
- Enquire about:
  - The patient's relationships with the family members
  - Their personalities

PERSONAL HISTORY

Early development

- Birth details – normal, caesarean (elective, emergency), any problems
- Mother–child relationship during first few years
- Development and milestones

Childhood temperament/behaviour

- Atmosphere at home
- Relationship between (and with) parents
- Relationship with siblings
- Presence of outside help, e.g. childminder, grandparents
- Temperament
- Emotional or behavioural disturbances, e.g. eating, sleeping, bed-wetting problems, nightmares, phobias, tantrums
- Antisocial behaviour – stealing, fighting

Illness and separation

- Severe illness/operations requiring hospitalization (patient, parent or sibling)
- Separation from parents, siblings – e.g. going into care
- Age of any changes/addition/loss to family and effects on patient

Education

- Number of schools
- Exams taken and passed
- Relationships with friends and teachers
- Problems with discipline, truanting
- Special needs

Occupation(s)

- Occupational history and length of posts
- Job satisfaction
- Relationships with work colleagues
- Redundancies, promotions

Psychosexual history

- Age of puberty, menarche, menopause
- First sexual interests/activity

- Intercourse with adults as a child
- Previous partner information/relationship details
- Libido, enjoyment of intercourse
- Pattern, frequency
- Influence of culture, religion

Marriage/partners

- Marital status – single, married, divorced, life partner
- Partner details – age, gender, occupation, health
- Relationship details – duration, how they met, any separations, trust issues

Children

- Ages
- Health
- Education, occupations
- Personalities
- Pregnancies – attitudes, mood, problems, birth details
- Miscarriages, terminations

Drugs and alcohol

- Smoking history
- Detailed alcohol history including first drink, quantity, addiction and misuse
- 'CAGE' questionnaire (see p. 19)

Forensic history

- Incidents involving the police
- Convictions, prison sentences, probation
- Lawsuits

Financial situation

- Source of income including benefits
- Financial worries

PREMORBID PERSONALITY

- Patient and informant (friends, relatives) accounts
- General outlook – cheerful, anxious, optimistic, controlled, extravagant
- Religion and other interests

MENTAL STATE EXAMINATION

Appearance and general behaviour

- Appearance – tidy, dishevelled, drawn, bizarre, appropriately dressed
- Manner – shy, anxious, friendly, reserved, suspicious, comment on rapport, e.g. good eye contact, appropriate responses
- Movements – restless, relaxed, tics, tremors, mannerisms, grimacing
- Is the patient responding to hallucinations?

Affect and mood

- Affect – 'emotional weather' – observed by doctor:
  - Flattened
  - Labile
  - Blunted
  - Incongruous
  - Reactive
  - Appropriate
- Mood – 'emotional climate' – patient's account:
  - Prevailing mood – happy, elated, sad, anxious, scared, angry
  - Feelings of guilt, hopelessness, blame
  - Capable of enjoyment/interest/concentration
- Beck's cognitive triad – ask patients how they feel about:
  - Themselves
  - The rest of the world
  - The future
- Suicide – interrogate the patient with regards to:
  - Ideas
  - Plans, method
  - Intent/preparation – have they put their affairs in order, made a will, planned a date, written notes?
- Risk:
  - To others
  - To themselves – thoughts of previous deliberate self-harm, through self-neglect
- Anxieties:
  - Fears, phobias or panic attacks
- Anger:
  - Intensity
  - Duration
  - Related to violence

BOX 1.13 SUICIDE RISK ASSESSMENT

A full psychiatric history should be obtained.

Specifically ask about:
- Thoughts around suicide
- Actions relating to it
- Plans (e.g. method)
- Letters written, affairs 'put in order'
- Previous attempts, or history of deliberate self-harm

Speech

- Form – relevant, coherent, spontaneous
- Rate – rapid, slow/retarded, interruptible, pressure of speech
- Quantity – elaborate, minimal, spontaneous, only in response to questions

- Volume – loud, soft
- Quality – normal, abnormal, e.g. dysphasic, slurred, stammering

Thought form

- Schizophrenic formal thought disorder:
  - Loose association between ideas
  - Tangential responses
  - Breakdown on syntax becoming incomprehensible
  - Jumbling of thoughts – 'word salad'
- Poverty of content – empty philosophizing
- Manic:
  - Flight of ideas (with connection)
  - Knight's move thinking
  - Neologisms (made-up words)
  - Puns
  - Rhymes and clangs

Thought content

- Preoccupations – fears, worries, phobias
- Obsessions:
  - Thoughts, images and impulses recognized by patient as absurd, often wants to resist them
  - Impede normal function
  - Associated with compulsive behaviours
- Abnormal beliefs and ideas:
  - Overvalued ideas, delusions
  - Firmly held beliefs contrary to everyday experience
  - Out of keeping with social, cultural and religious beliefs
  - *Not* amenable to argument
- Delusions:
  - Primary – arise spontaneously, may be preceded by delusional or 'odd' mood, subdivided into:
    - Delusional – attribution of new meaning to normal object
    - Autochthonous – arising without apparent cause
  - Secondary – arise from other experiences, e.g.:
    - Mood disorders
    - Perceptual disturbances
    - Delusions
    - Passivity
  - Content may involve:
    - Jealousy, sex or love
    - Grandiose, religious or fantastic ideas
    - Ill health, persecution or nihilism
    - Possession of thought, e.g. through insertion, broadcasting or withdrawal
- Abnormal experiences and perceptions:
  - Hallucinations – false perception perceived in external space (no external stimulus)
  - Pseudo-hallucinations – internal stimulus

- ○ Perceptual disorders – auditory, visual, olfactory, gustatory, tactile or derealization, depersonalization, *déjà vu, jamais vu*
- ○ Illusions – abnormal or distorted perceptions of external reality
- Cognitive state, i.e. Mini-Mental State Examination (MMSE – see p. 98)
- Insight – are they aware:
  - ○ Why this started?
  - ○ That they are unwell?
  - ○ What the causes might be?
  - ○ What treatment they might need and what the prognosis is?

Examination

CARDIOVASCULAR SYSTEM

CARDIOVASCULAR EXAMINATION

INTRODUCTION

- Explain the procedure
- Ask about painful areas
- Request permission
- Position patient sitting at 45°
- Expose from waist up

INSPECTION

General

- Cyanotic, plethoric, pale
- Tachypnoea
- Scars on chest – midline sternotomy, lateral thoracotomy
- Pacemaker
- Visible impulses
- Scars on leg from previous CABG vein harvest

Hands

- Capillary refill and temperature
- Colour – cyanosis, pale
- Nails – clubbing, splinter haemorrhages, koilonychia
- Janeway lesions (red macules on palms)
- Osler's nodes (painful nodules in the finger pulps)
- Tar staining

Pulses

- Radial – rate and rhythm
- Brachial – character (paradoxus, alternans, collapsing, slow rising – see Box 2.1), volume

- Compare arms – different volume, delay (aortic arch deformity)
- Blood pressure

BOX 2.1 ABNORMAL PULSE CHARACTERS

- Paradoxus – diminished pulse on inspiration, e.g. tamponade, obstructive lung disease
- Alternans – varies with every other beat, e.g. left ventricular systolic impairment
- Collapsing (waterhammer) – aortic regurgitation
- Slow rising – aortic stenosis

Jugular venous pressure (JVP) – see page 30

- Should have double waveform and be non-palpable
- Height – measured vertically above sternal angle, approximately 3–4 cm
- Waveform constitutes a and v, as well as x and y descents
- Hepatojugular reflux confirms identification of JVP with concurrent rise
- Interpreting the JVP:
  - Raised – (right) heart failure
  - Reduced – hypovolaemia
  - Cannon waves – complete heart block
  - Absent 'a' waves – atrial fibrillation
  - Large 'v' waves – tricuspid regurgitation

Face

- Central cyanosis – lips, tongue
- Malar flush (mitral stenosis)
- Tongue – smooth, 'beefy'
- Eyes – anaemia, xanthelasma, small Argyll Robertson pupil, corneal arcus

PALPATION

Apex beat

- Position patient at 45°, lean to left lateral position, if needed, to accentuate impulse
- Should be located in fifth intercostal space, mid-clavicular line
- Displacement may be due to dilatation of the left ventricle
- Character may be changed in left ventricular hypertrophy (thrusting)

Heaves

- Use ball of hand on the left sternal edge (for right ventricular heave)
- Use ulnar border of left hand to second intercostal space bilaterally for pulmonary and aortic dilation

BOX 2.2 INTERPRETING COMMON MURMURS

- Aortic stenosis – ejection systolic, best heard at upper right sternal edge in expiration, radiating to the neck with slow rising pulse
- Aortic regurgitation – early diastolic murmur, collapsing pulse, nail bed pulsation and visible carotids (Corrigan's sign), heard best at lower left sternal edge, leaning forward
- Mitral regurgitation – pansystolic murmur heard loudest over apex, in left lateral position in expiration, radiating into axilla
- Mitral stenosis – diastolic, best heard over apex with bell of stethoscope

AUSCULTATION

- Listen and time heart sounds with carotid pulse
- Listen to the four regions in turn (see Fig. 2.1)
  - Apex (mitral region)
    - Turn to the left lateral position, ask for a deep breath in, out and to hold it while listening with the bell
    - A tapping/diastolic rumble from mitral stenosis may be heard
    - Move back to the recumbent position and listen over the same area with the diaphragm
  - Left upper sternal edge (pulmonary region)
    - Note physiological splitting of first sound
  - Left lower sternal edge (tricuspid region)

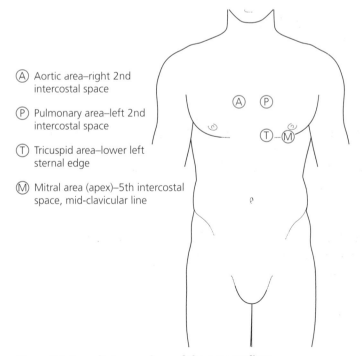

Ⓐ Aortic area–right 2nd intercostal space

Ⓟ Pulmonary area–left 2nd intercostal space

Ⓣ Tricuspid area–lower left sternal edge

Ⓜ Mitral area (apex)–5th intercostal space, mid-clavicular line

Figure 2.1 Auscultatory regions of the praecordium

- ♦ Lean patient forwards, request deep breath in and out, then hold, listening for aortic regurgitation with diaphragm
    - ○ Base, upper right sternal edge (aortic region)
        - ♦ High frequency – use diaphragm
        - ♦ Listen for aortic stenosis (radiates to carotids)
- Listen over carotids
    - ○ Bruits, aortic stenosis radiation
- Listen for femoral, renal bruits, 'pistol-shot' over femorals
- Listen (and percuss) lung bases for bi-basal crepitations of pulmonary oedema

---

BOX 2.3 MURMUR MANOEUVRES

- Leaning left – makes mitral stenosis murmur louder
- Leaning forward – makes aortic regurgitation murmur louder
- Breathing in – makes murmurs on the right side louder
- Breathing out – makes left-sided murmurs louder

EXTRAS

- Complete examination by palpating for abdominal aortic aneurysm, enlarged liver (typically smooth, pulsatile hepatomegaly in right heart failure) and peripheral pulses (e.g. radio-femoral delay)
- Look for peripheral/sacral oedema
- Consider
    - ○ Taking the patient for a walk to assess exercise tolerance
    - ○ Examining the fundi for hypertensive/diabetic/endocarditis changes

TESTS

- Bloods tests, e.g. haemoglobin for anaemia with prosthetic aortic valves, inflammatory markers in endocarditis
- Electrocardiogram (ECG) – evidence of arrhythmias, hypertrophy
- Temperature – raised in infective endocarditis
- Dipstick urine – for haematuria in endocarditis
- Chest X-ray (posteroanterior) – to assess size of cardiac shadow, presence of pulmonary oedema
- Echocardiogram – to assess structure and function

JUGULAR VENOUS PRESSURE

Jugular venous pressure (JVP) analysis provides useful information about a patient's cardiovascular state.

It essentially represents a manometer in direct communication with the right atrium, and therefore can give information about venous pressure as well as valvular function.

OBSERVING THE JUGULAR VENOUS PRESSURE

This is best done with:

- The patient at 45°
- The patient's head turned slightly to the left

Locate the internal jugular vein as it passes:

- Between the inferior heads of the sternocleidomastoid muscle
- Upwards behind the angle of the jaw, to the earlobe

The JVP corresponds to the **vertical** distance the double pulsation is visible above the sternal angle. It is considered raised if it is above 3–4 cmH_2O.

BOX 2.4 DIFFERENTIATING BETWEEN VENOUS AND ARTERIAL PULSATION IN THE NECK

	JVP	**Carotid**
Waveform	Double pulse	Single pulse
Palpation	Not palpable	Pulse palpable
Hepatojugular reflux	Rises	No change
Obliteration with finger	Possible	Not possible

JVP WAVEFORM

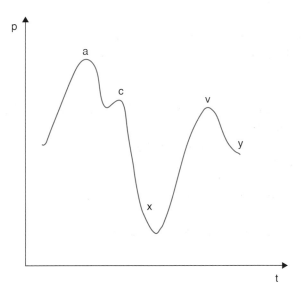

Figure 2.2 Classic JVP waveform

A typical waveform consists of:

- An 'a' wave – this corresponds to atrial contraction
- A 'c' wave – this corresponds to tricuspid valve closure
- An 'x' descent – this corresponds to the atrium relaxing and then filling against closed tricuspid, to wave 'v'

- A 'v' wave – this corresponds to a tense atrium filling against a closed tricuspid valve
- 'y' descent – this corresponds to emptying of the atrium through an open tricuspid

ABNORMAL JVPs

There are several abnormalities that the JVP can exhibit:

- Raised JVP: right-sided heart failure, superior vena cava obstruction (+ absent pulsation)
- Cannon waves: occur when atrium contracts against closed tricuspid, e.g. heart block
- Large 'a' waves: pulmonary or tricuspid stenosis
- Absent 'a' waves: atrial fibrillation
- Large 'v' waves: tricuspid regurgitation
- Deep 'x' and 'y' descent: constrictive pericarditis/tamponade (also have JVP rise on inspiration and 'fixed' plateau)

INVESTIGATIONS

ECG, chest X-ray and echocardiogram will confirm or assess cardiac status if any of the above are noted on examination.

HEART FAILURE

Heart failure can affect predominantly the left, the right, or both sides of the heart, giving rise to differing symptoms and signs.

Cardiac failure can be classified as high (increased tissue demand) or low (normal tissue requirements) output in nature, with the latter being far more common.

LOW-OUTPUT HEART FAILURE

BOX 2.5 CAUSES OF LOW-OUTPUT HEART FAILURE

- Pressure overload, e.g. hypertension, aortic stenosis
- Volume overload, e.g. aortic regurgitation, sepsis
- Arrhythmias, e.g. complete heart block, supraventricular tachycardia
- Systolic failure, e.g. myocardial infarction, myocarditis
- Diastolic failure, e.g. restrictive cardiomyopathy, tamponade

---

HISTORY

- Dyspnoea (especially on exertion)
- Orthopnoea
- Paroxysmal nocturnal dyspnoea (PND)
- Palpitations
- Peripheral oedema

INSPECTION

- General:
    - ○ Oedema: ankle, lower limb, sacral, anasarca (generalized)
    - ○ Weight loss
- Pulse:
    - ○ Tachycardia
    - ○ Arrhythmia, e.g. atrial fibrillation, complete heart block
    - ○ Pulsus alternans (alternate strong and weak pulse)
- JVP:
    - ○ Raised in right-sided (or congestive) cardiac failure

PALPATION

- Displaced apex beat
- Left ventricular heave

AUSCULTATION

- Heart:
    - ○ Third heart sound (S3 gallop rhythm)
    - ○ Loud P2 (right-sided)
- Lung:
    - ○ Bi-basal crepitations, crackles or wheeze
    - ○ Pleural effusion

BOX 2.6 SIGNS OF HEART FAILURE

Congestive heart failure will present with a combination of signs listed below.

Left-sided:
- Dyspnoea
- Bi-basal crepitations
- Abnormal pulse e.g. alternans
- Cardiomegaly

Right-sided:
- Raised JVP
- Loud P2
- S3 gallop rhythm
- Peripheral oedema
- Hepatomegaly, ascites, pleural effusions

INVESTIGATIONS

- *Blood tests*: full blood count (FBC) – anaemia; urea and electrolytes (U&E) – concomitant renal failure, liver function tests – for evidence of congestive liver disease
- *Arterial blood gases*: hypoxia
- *ECG*: arrhythmias, left ventricular hypertrophy
- *Chest X-ray*: cardiomegaly, bilateral hilar pulmonary infiltrates, upper lobe diversion, Kerley B lines, pleural effusion
- *Echocardiogram*: assess and quantify ventricular and valvular dysfunction and/or reduced myocardial wall movement
- *Angiography*: to detect (and treat) potential causes, e.g. coronary artery disease

TREATMENT

- Lifestyle changes, e.g. optimal nutrition, salt restriction
- Treat underlying cause, e.g. valve replacement
- Drugs, e.g. angiotensin-converting enzyme (ACE) inhibitors, β-blockers, spironolactone, diuretics, nitrates
- Heart transplantation (in very selected cases)

HIGH-OUTPUT CARDIAC FAILURE

- This is far rarer than low-output cardiac failure
- Involves normal or high cardiac output
- Causes include pregnancy, hyperthyroidism, Paget's disease

AORTIC MURMURS

Aortic murmurs commonly occur in clinical examinations. They include aortic stenosis, aortic regurgitation or mixed valve disease.

AORTIC STENOSIS

Inspection

- Tachypnoea
- Midline sternotomy scar (after valve replacement)
- Pulse:
  - Slow-rising
  - Small volume
- Blood pressure:
  - Narrow pulse pressure
- Jugular venous pressure:
  - Normal

Palpation

- Displaced apex beat and heave (depending on degree of any failure)
- Systolic thrill over carotids and right upper sternal edge (aortic area)

BOX 2.7 ASSESSING SEVERITY/INDICATIONS FOR SURGERY

- Symptoms: exertional dyspnoea, chest pain, syncopal attacks
- Pressure gradient: systolic gradient across valve of >50–60 mmHg
- Valve area: less than 1.0 cm^2

Auscultation

- Ejection systolic murmur loudest at the right upper sternal edge, radiating to the carotids
- Louder in expiration (as left-sided lesion) and on sitting forward
- Quiet aortic second sound (or inaudible)

- Ejection 'click' (bicuspid valve)
- Bi-basal crepitations (with failing left ventricle)

Investigations

- ECG
- Chest X-ray
- Echocardiogram (transthoracic)
- Cardiac catheterization

BOX 2.8 CAUSES OF AORTIC STENOSIS

Congenital
Acquired:
- Bicuspid aortic valve
- Degenerative calcification
- Rheumatic heart disease

Treatment

- Surgical replacement of aortic valve
- Percutaneous aortic valve replacement (if patient unfit)
- Palliative

AORTIC SCLEROSIS

- Caused by senile degeneration
- Exhibits an ejection systolic murmur
- Normal S_2, no click
- Normal pulses
- NO thrills or heaves
- NO significant murmur radiation to the carotids
- NOT associated with left ventricular outflow tract obstruction

AORTIC REGURGITATION

Inspection

- Quincke's sign – visible nail bed pulsation
- De Musset's sign – visible head titubation
- Corrigan's sign – visible neck pulsation (carotids)
- Tachypnoea
- Midline sternotomy scar
- Pulse:
  - Regular (usually)
  - Collapsing (waterhammer) pulse
- Blood pressure:
  - Widened pulse pressure (depending on severity)
- Jugular venous pressure:
  - Normal (Corrigan's sign may be noted – see above)

Palpation

- Sustained, displaced apex beat

Auscultation

- Early diastolic murmur (high-pitched)
  - Louder in expiration and on sitting forward
- Austin–Flint murmur (mid-diastole at apex) may be heard – due to vibration of the anterior mitral valve leaflet by regurgitant jet
- Bi-basal crepitations (with failing left ventricle)
- Traube's sign – pistol shot heard over femoral artery
- Duroziez's sign – murmur heard over femoral artery on compression with a stethoscope

---

BOX 2.9 CAUSES OF AORTIC REGURGITATION

Congenital
Acquired:

- Hypertensive disease
- Infective endocarditis
- Rheumatic heart disease
- Connective tissue diseases, e.g. Marfan's syndrome, ankylosing spondylitis

---

Investigations

- ECG
- Chest X-ray
- Echocardiogram (transthoracic)
- Cardiac catheterization

Treatment

- Vasodilators to prolong time to deterioration
- Replace valve before severe left ventricular dysfunction occurs (assess with serial echocardiograms)

MIXED AORTIC VALVE DISEASE

- Patients may present with mixed symptoms and signs of stenosis and regurgitant murmurs
- It is not uncommon for them to have mixed aortic valve disease and the signs should be presented as such, with an attempt to specify the predominant lesion, and why

MITRAL MURMURS

Mitral murmurs also commonly occur in clinical examinations. They include mitral stenosis, mitral regurgitation or mixed valve disease.

Rheumatic heart disease is the most common cause of mitral stenosis, but is now rare in the developed world.

MITRAL STENOSIS

Inspection

- Malar flush (mitral facies)
- Peripheral cyanosis
- Tachypnoea
- Midline or left lateral/axillary thoracotomy scar
- If valvular disease is severe and pulmonary hypertension develops there may be signs of right-sided heart failure (peripheral oedema, loud P2, pulsatile liver)
- Pulse:
  - Typically irregularly irregular (i.e. atrial fibrillation [AF]), less commonly sinus rhythm
  - Small volume
- Blood pressure:
  - Normal
- Jugular venous pressure:
  - Normal or raised in presence of right heart failure

Palpation

- Undisplaced, tapping apex beat – S_1 – (unless in left ventricular failure)
- Left parasternal heave

Auscultation

- Loud first heart sound
- Loud P2
- Opening snap
- Mid-diastolic rumbling murmur heard best at the apex in left lateral position
- Murmur is more pronounced after exercise (e.g. ask patient to walk up and down ward quickly)
- A Graham Steell murmur may also be present (early diastolic murmur of pulmonary regurgitation)
- Bilateral crepitations consistent with left ventricular failure

Investigations

- ECG – AF, P mitrale, right ventricular hypertrophy
- Chest X-ray – large left atrium, calcification of valve, pulmonary oedema
- Echocardiogram (transthoracic) – opening <1 cm^2/m^2 body surface area
- Cardiac catheterization

BOX 2.10 CAUSES OF MITRAL STENOSIS

Congenital
Acquired:
- Rheumatic heart disease
- Connective tissue diseases, e.g. rheumatoid arthritis, systemic lupus erythematosus

Treatment

- Anticoagulation for AF
- Surgery or percutaneous valvuloplasty is indicated if the patient develops:
  - Pulmonary oedema (without alternative cause)
  - Significant symptoms
  - Emboli and/or haemoptysis

MITRAL REGURGITATION

Inspection

- Tachypnoea
- Midline or left lateral/axillary thoracotomy scar
- Signs of left-sided heart failure (e.g. pulmonary oedema)
- Pulse:
  - Regular or AF
- Blood pressure:
  - Normal
- Jugular venous pressure:
  - Normal

Palpation

- Thrusting, displaced apex beat
- Systolic thrill
- Left parasternal heave (if severe mitral regurgitation)

Auscultation

- Quiet S1
- Pan-systolic murmur
  - Loudest at the apex, radiates to the axilla
  - Heard loudest in the left lateral position
- Presence of a third heart sound (severe mitral regurgitation)
- Widened splitting of S2 or fourth heart sound
- Bilateral crepitations consistent with left ventricular failure

---

BOX 2.11 CAUSES OF MITRAL REGURGITATION

Congenital
Acquired:
- Degenerative
- Hypertensive disease, i.e. severe left ventricular dilatation
- Infective endocarditis
- Rheumatic heart disease
- Mitral valve prolapse
- Connective tissue diseases, e.g. Marfan's syndrome, ankylosing spondylitis
- Papillary muscle rupture, e.g. post myocardial infarction

Investigations

- ECG
- Chest X-ray – cardiomegaly
- Echocardiogram (transthoracic)
- Cardiac catheterization

Treatment

- Treatment of heart failure
- Anticoagulation for AF
- Valve repair or replacement if any of:
  - Severe symptoms
  - Left ventricular failure
  - Left ventricular dilatation

MIXED MITRAL VALVE DISEASE

- Patients may present with mixed symptoms and signs of stenosis and regurgitant murmurs
- It is not uncommon for them to have mixed mitral valve disease and the signs should be presented as such, with an attempt to specify the predominant lesion, and why

BACTERIAL/INFECTIVE ENDOCARDITIS

Bacterial endocarditis is an infection of the endothelial lining of the heart. Approximately halfiz of all cases occur on structurally normal valves and are secondary to a bacteraemia, e.g. urethral catheter insertion, dental procedures. It is most commonly caused by viridians type *Streptococcus* (~ 50% of cases) but other organisms include *Enterococcus, Staphylococcus aureus, Coxiella* and fungi.

HISTORY

- Fever/rigors
- Weight loss/anorexia
- Lethargy/malaise
- Rash

EXAMINATION

Patients may exhibit signs of the four main clinical manifestations of bacterial endocarditis:

- New heart murmur
- Vasculitic, e.g. Osler's nodes
- Embolic, e.g. stroke
- Infective, e.g. fever

INSPECTION

General

- Pyrexia
- Petechiae/vasculitic rash
- Arthritis
- Signs of stroke – see page 102

Hands

- Clubbing
- Splinter haemorrhages (>2)
- Osler's nodes (tender nodules of the fingertip pulps)
- Janeway lesions (non-tender erythematous macules on the palm/sole)

Pulse

- Normal or tachycardic
- May be collapsing if aortic valve involved and regurgitant

JVP

- Raised in the presence of congestive heart failure
- Large 'v' waves with tricuspid disease/regurgitation

Eyes

- Roth's spots – white retinal exudates, surrounded by haemorrhage

PALPATION

- Normal or relating to acute valvular or cardiac failure (e.g. displaced apex)
- Splenomegaly

AUSCULTATION

- New murmur, e.g. mitral or tricuspid (right-sided) in intravenous drug users
- Bi-basal crepitations (if in heart failure)

BOX 2.12 DUKE CRITERIA FOR DIAGNOSING INFECTIVE ENDOCARDITIS

Three major, one major and three minor or five minor for diagnosis.
Major criteria:

- Positive blood culture (two or more separate cultures, or persistently positive, i.e. >12 hours apart, or three or majority of four positive separate samples)
- Endocardial involvement (positive echocardiogram for vegetation, abscess or prosthetic valve dehiscence or new valvular regurgitation)

Minor criteria:

- Positive blood culture (not fulfilling above criteria)
- Positive echocardiogram (not fulfilling above criteria)
- High fever (>38°C)
- Predisposition (intravenous drug user, known cardiac lesion)
- Immunological or vascular phenomena (glomerulonephritis, Janeway lesions)

INVESTIGATIONS

- Blood tests, e.g. to assess anaemia, inflammatory markers (high erythrocyte sedimentation rate [ESR]), renal failure, serological tests for fastidious organisms, e.g. *Legionella*, rheumatoid factor (becomes positive, then negative when treated)
- Blood cultures (at least three sets) – different sites, different times (aseptic technique is key)
- Urinalysis – microscopic haematuria
- ECG – may show conduction delay (PR interval prolongation)
- Chest X-ray – signs of heart failure
- Echocardiogram – transthoracic ± transoesophageal (see Box 2.12)

TREATMENT

(Depending on organism)

- Antibiotics, e.g. benzylpenicillin, gentamicin
- Surgery, e.g. valve replacement

COMPLICATIONS

- Anaemia
- Renal failure
- Stroke
- Heart failure
- Death ~6–30 per cent (depending on organism)

PROSTHETIC VALVES

Prosthetic valves are common in examinations owing to the wealth of clinical signs and the lengthy discussion which they can provide.

Essentially you may be expected to:

- Recognize a prosthesis is present and its position
- Offer a diagnosis with supporting evidence
- Comment on how well the valve appears to be working
- Discuss the issues of anticoagulation and endocarditis

INSPECTION

- Scars:
  - Midline sternotomy
  - Lateral thoracotomy
  - Saphenous harvest (lower legs) – if accompanied by a midline sternotomy scar, this may be explained by coronary artery bypass graft surgery
- Bruising (may be significant if over-anticoagulated)
- Stigmata of infective endocarditis (see p. 39)

Note: While examining listen carefully for a mechanical 'ticking' from a metallic prosthesis.

PALPATION

- Normal
- Pulse:
  - Normal (unless valve failing, e.g. collapsing pulse of aortic incompetence)
- If valve failing signs such as displaced apex might be present

AUSCULTATION

Aortic valve replacement

- Normal first heart sound
- Opening (ejection) click
- Ejection systolic murmur (normal flow murmur over valve)
- Metallic second heart sound (click)
- Addition of a collapsing pulse and early diastolic murmur would signify valve incompetence and failure

Mitral valve replacement

- Metallic click of the first heart sound
- Normal second heart sound
- Opening (diastolic) click
- Mid-diastolic murmur (seldom heard flow murmur)
- Addition of a pan-systolic murmur may suggest valve incompetence

Note:

- Both valves may have been replaced
- Tissue grafts may exhibit normal heart sounds or mild flow murmurs only

---

BOX 2.13 TISSUE AND MECHANICAL PROSTHETIC VALVES

	Tissue	**Mechanical**
Anticoagulation	Not required	Required lifelong
Lifespan	Limited: 8–10 years	Long-lasting
Complications	Calcification	Thromboembolism, endocarditis

INVESTIGATIONS

- Blood tests, e.g. haemoglobin for anaemia, inflammatory markers for endocarditis, clotting screen to monitor warfarin treatment
- Echocardiogram to assess valve function (leakage predisposes to infective endocarditis)

COMPLICATIONS

- Thromboembolic event
- Infective endocarditis
- Leakage, failure and heart failure
- Haemorrhage (due to over-anticoagulation)
- Haemolytic anaemia (aortic valves)

RESPIRATORY SYSTEM

RESPIRATORY EXAMINATION

INTRODUCTION

- Explain the examination
- Ask about painful areas
- Request permission and offer chaperone
- Position patient on couch, sitting at 45°
- Expose appropriately (ideally remove clothes from waist up)

INSPECTION

General

- Note any equipment present
  - ○ O_2 mask or nasal cannulae
  - ○ Inhalers, spacers or sputum pot (examine inside) nearby
- Colour: pink or blue in the face (see below)
- Shortness of breath
  - ○ Respiratory rate (measured surreptitiously so as not to influence)
  - ○ Accessory muscle use
  - ○ Bracing against bed
  - ○ Nasal flaring, pursed lips
- Chest shape
  - ○ Pectus carinatum (pigeon-shaped) – common after childhood chronic respiratory disease
  - ○ Pectus excavatum (funnel-shaped) – developmental defect
  - ○ Barrel (increased anteroposterior diameter) – emphysema
  - ○ Thoracic kyphoscoliosis – reduced ventilatory capacity/increased work of breathing
- Chest wall movement
- Scars from biopsy, thoracoscopy, pneumonectomy, transplants

Hands

- Clubbing, hypertrophic pulmonary osteoarthropathy
- Cyanosis, tar staining
- Wasting of the small muscles of the hand (lung cancer invading brachial plexus)
- Asterixis (CO_2 retention flap), fine tremor (from β_2-agonists)

Pulse

- Rate and rhythm
- Character (bounding in CO_2 retention)
- Blood pressure

BOX 2.14 CAUSES OF CLUBBING (SEE P. 52)

Congenital

Respiratory:
- Bronchial malignancy
- Idiopathic pulmonary fibrosis (IPF)
- Suppurative lung diseases:
  - empyema
  - lung abscess
  - bronchiectasis
  - cystic fibrosis

Cardiac:
- atrial myxoma
- bacterial endocarditis
- cyanotic heart disease

Abdominal:
- cirrhosis
- Crohn's disease
- ulcerative colitis
- coeliac disease

Face

- Pink, blue, lip pursing
- Eyes: pallor (anaemia)
- Horner's syndrome: ptosis and constricted pupil (invasion of sympathetic chain by Pancoast's apical tumour and ipsilateral hand wasting)
- Tongue: central cyanosis, oral candidiasis from steroid inhaler use

Neck

- JVP – raised, prominent v wave of tricuspid regurgitation (e.g. right-sided heart failure due to cor pulmonale)
- Lymphadenopathy
- Tracheal deviation, tug (e.g. tension pneumothorax)

PALPATION

- Right ventricular heave (secondary to cor pulmonale)
- Expansion – front and back (asymmetric after pneumonectomy)
- Tactile vocal fremitus in all areas – ask patient to say '99' and feel with ulnar aspect of hands (reduced in effusion, increased in consolidation – see Table 2.1)

Table 2.1 Common clinical findings

Pathology	Expansion	Air entry	Vocal resonance	Percussion
Pneumothorax	Reduced	Reduced	Reduced	Hyperresonant
Consolidation	Reduced	Reduced	Increased	Dull
Effusion	Reduced	Reduced	Reduced	Stony dull

PERCUSSION

- All areas, comparing one side to the other, including clavicles
- Consolidation: bronchial breathing and crepitations may be present
- Effusion: an area of bronchial breathing may be heard above the effusion

AUSCULTATION

- All areas (including right axilla)

- Comment on sounds: equal, vesicular (normal)/bronchial (coarse), added sounds
  - Crackles (crepitations) – may be cleared on coughing
  - Rubs – like 'stepping on fresh snow'
  - Wheeze – inspiratory/expiratory/mono or polyphonic
- Vocal resonance: ask the patient to say '99' – listen with bell
  - Increased resonance in the presence of consolidation
  - Reduced with effusions
- Whispering pectoriloquy: ask patient to whisper '111' – listen with diaphragm – replicates vocal resonance

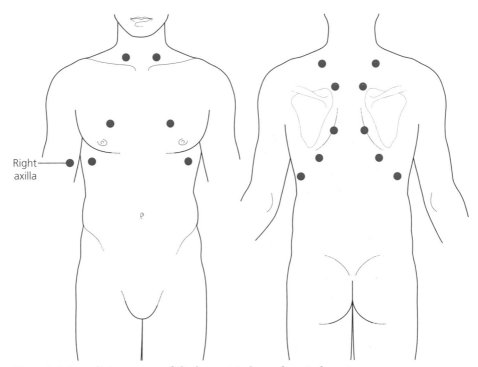

Figure 2.3 Auscultatory areas of the lung: anterior and posterior

Tests

- Full set of blood tests
- Peak expiratory flow rate (PEFR) ± formal spirometry
- Oxygen saturations
- Arterial blood gas
- Sputum microscopy and culture
- Chest X-ray (± high-resolution computed tomography (CT) scan)
- Temperature

CHRONIC OBSTRUCTIVE PULMONARY DISEASE

This common disease invariably arises in later life usually as a result of chronic cigarette smoking.

Complications include exacerbations requiring hospitalization, recurrent pneumonia, pneumothoraces, bronchial carcinoma, pulmonary hypertension and heart failure.

HISTORY

- Shortness of breath
- Recurrent cough
- Sputum production
- Wheezing
- Lethargy
- Weight loss

FAMILY HISTORY

- α_1-antitrypsin deficiency (lower zone emphysema and liver disease)

SOCIAL HISTORY

- Significant smoking history
- Occupational exposure to coal mining or heavy metals
- Exposure to pollution

EXAMINATION

General

- Inhalers, nebulizers, oxygen or sputum pots by bed
- Cachectic

Hands

- Tar-stained fingers
- Peripheral cyanosis
- Bounding pulse (CO_2 retention)
- Asterixis (CO_2 retention flap)
- Clubbing from related disease, e.g. bronchial carcinoma, not a feature of chronic obstructive pulmonary disease (COPD) alone

Neck

- Raised JVP with visible v wave (sign of tricuspid regurgitation, often secondary to pulmonary hypertension)
- Reduced cricoid to suprasternal notch distance (hyperinflation)

Face

- Central cyanosis
- Use of accessory muscles, e.g. nasal flaring
- Plethoric
- Pursed-lip breathing

Chest

- Respiratory rate
- Accessory muscle use, e.g. indrawing of intercostal muscles
- Chest shape, often barrel-shaped – increased anteroposterior diameter

- Equal movement
- Scars

PALPATION

- Expansion – may be reduced
- Percussion note – may be hyperresonant throughout with hyperexpansion including loss of usual dullness over the heart and liver
- Tactile vocal fremitus – may isolate an area of consolidation (infection, carcinoma)

AUSCULTATION

- Heart: loud P2, tricuspid regurgitation (signs of pulmonary hypertension – see Box 2.15)
- Lungs: reduced breath sounds throughout added sounds: wheeze, crackles (may change on coughing)

BOX 2.15 SIGNS OF PULMONARY HYPERTENSION

- Raised JVP with prominent v wave
- Ankle ± sacral oedema
- Loud P2
- Tricuspid regurgitation
- Pulmonary regurgitation
- Pulsatile and tender enlarged liver

INVESTIGATIONS

- Full blood count (may be anaemic or polycythaemic)
- Arterial blood gases (may be hypoxic, hypercapnic)
- Sputum microscopy and culture (concurrent pneumonia, pneumothorax)
- Chest X-ray (hyperinflation, flattened diaphragm, bullae)
- ECG (right axis deviation and bundle branch block, p pulmonale)
- Spirometry (obstructive picture: FEV_1/FVC ratio <70 per cent)

TREATMENT

- Smoking cessation and pulmonary rehabilitation
- Dietetic input to treat respiratory cachexia
- Inhalers: bronchodilators (e.g. salbutamol/salmeterol), antimuscarinics (e.g. ipratropium/tiotropium), steroids (e.g. fluticasone)
- Oral steroid therapy to treat exacerbations
- Long-term oxygen therapy and home nebulizers
- Lung volume reduction surgery or transplant in very selected cases

ASTHMA

Asthma is defined as reversible airways inflammation and narrowing, causing wheeze, shortness of breath and cough.

HISTORY

- Recurrent attacks of:
  - Shortness of breath
  - Wheezing
- Cough – worse at night and early mornings
- Atopy – hayfever, eczema
- Allergies – dust, animals, pollen, mould
- Occupational exposure
- Triggers – cigarette smoke, exercise, cold weather

INSPECTION

During attacks patient may present with:

- Shortness of breath – may be unable to complete sentences
- Use of accessory muscles
- Cyanosis (life-threatening sign)

EXAMINATION

This is often normal in between attacks.

- Pulse:
  - Tachycardia
  - Pulsus paradoxus (fall of >10 mmHg in systolic blood pressure during inspiration – sign of acute severe asthma compromising venous return)
- Chest:
  - Tachypnoea
  - Widespread polyphonic expiratory (and inspiratory) wheeze
  - Prolonged expiratory phase
  - Difficulty completing sentences
  - Silent chest (life-threatening sign – see Box 2.16)

INVESTIGATIONS

- PEFR
- Full blood tests (to rule out underlying infection)
- Sputum analysis
- Pulse oximetry
- Arterial blood gases if suspected severe asthma
- Chest X-ray if suspected infection/pneumothorax

TREATMENT

- High flow oxygen
- Oral steroids unless patient unable to swallow
- Nebulized salbutamol (or intravenous or inhaled via spacer)
- Ipratropium bromide (nebulized)
- Magnesium sulphate (intravenous)
- Consider aminophylline if failing to respond to all other therapies (do not load if already on regular aminophylline)
- Early referral to intensivist for non-invasive or invasive ventilation

BOX 2.16 ASSESSING SEVERITY OF ADULT ASTHMA ATTACKS (BRITISH THORACIC SOCIETY GUIDELINES)

Moderate exacerbation:
- Increasing symptoms
- PEFR >50–75 per cent best or predicted
- No features of acute severe asthma

Acute severe – any one of:
- PEFR 33–50 per cent best or predicted
- Respiratory rate ≥25/minute
- Heart rate ≥110/minute
- Inability to complete sentences in one breath

Life-threatening – a patient with severe asthma and any one of:
- PEFR <33 per cent best or predicted
- SpO_2 <92 per cent
- PaO_2 <8 kPa
- Normal $PaCO_2$ (4.6–6.0 kPa)
- Silent chest
- Cyanosis
- Poor respiratory effort
- Bradycardia, arrhythmia, hypotension
- Exhaustion, coma, confusion

Near-fatal
- Raised $PaCO_2$ and/or requiring mechanical ventilation with raised inflation pressures

IDIOPATHIC PULMONARY FIBROSIS

Previously known as fibrosing alveolitis, idiopathic pulmonary fibrosis (IPF) represents a spectrum of inflammatory fibrosis ranging from the more severe fibrotic usual interstitial pneumonitis (UIP) to the inflammatory desquamative interstitial pneumonitis (DIP).

HISTORY

- Progressive shortness of breath, usually over several years
- Non-productive (dry) cough
- Medical history of connective tissue disease (see Box 2.17)
- History of exposure to animals, plants, occupational dusts (see Box 2.17)

EXAMINATION

- Over 5 per cent of fibrosis is asymptomatic and an incidental finding on examination
- Clubbing (in over 50 per cent of patients with IPF)
- Bilateral fine ('showers' of) end-expiratory crackles
- Central or peripheral cyanosis (if severe)
- Respiratory distress

- Right-sided heart failure (cor pulmonale)
  - Prominent v wave in JVP
  - Right ventricular heave
  - Loud P2
  - Tricuspid and/or pulmonary regurgitation
  - Hepatomegaly
  - Peripheral oedema

INVESTIGATIONS

- Arterial blood gases
- Pulmonary function tests (to assess severity) – restrictive defect (see p. 231)
- Chest X-ray: diffuse interstitial 'honeycomb' shadowing
- High resolution CT scan
- Bronchoalveolar lavage analysis
- Lung biopsy

BOX 2.17 CAUSES OF PULMONARY FIBROSIS

Extrinsic allergic alveolitis
(organic dust disease):
- Bird fancier's lung
- Farmer's lung
- Malt worker's lung

Pneumoconioses
(inorganic dust disease):
- Coal worker's lung
- Silicosis
- Asbestosis

Connective tissue diseases:
- Ankylosing spondylitis
- Systemic lupus erythematosus
- Rheumatoid arthritis
- Systemic sclerosis

Drugs:
- Methotrexate
- Amiodarone
- Nitrofurantoin
- Gold

Others:
- Sarcoidosis
- Radiotherapy
- Pulmonary vasculitis

TREATMENT

- High-dose steroids
- Immunosuppression (e.g. with azathioprine)
- Supportive treatment:
  - Long-term oxygen therapy
  - Antibiotics (for infection)
  - Diuretics for fluid retention in cor pulmonale
- Lung transplantation for selected patients

BRONCHIAL CARCINOMA (LUNG CANCER)

Bronchial carcinoma refers to any malignant lesion of the respiratory tree epithelium. It often presents late and the majority are non-resectable.

Over 38 000 people are diagnosed with lung cancer each year in the UK.

HISTORY

The following symptoms and signs often herald a typically late presentation. Coexisting lung pathology, e.g. COPD, may mask symptoms.

- Cough, sputum production, haemoptysis
- Shortness of breath, chest pain (may be pleuritic)
- Weight loss, anorexia and tiredness
- Pneumonia (secondary infection distal to malignant obstruction)
- Clubbing and hypertrophic osteoarthropathy
- Neuropathy or myopathy
- Pancoast's tumour – apical tumour affecting sympathetic trunk (Horner's syndrome) ± brachial plexus
- Hoarse voice – recurrent laryngeal nerve invasion
- Superior vena cava obstruction
- Dysphagia and broncho-oesophageal fistula
- Endocrine syndromes
  - ○ Parathyroid hormone-related peptide (PTHrP) producing small-cell carcinomas resulting in hypercalcaemia
  - ○ Ectopic adrenocorticotropic hormone (ACTH) production causing Cushing's syndrome (see p. 151)

RISK FACTORS

- Cigarette smoking
- Air pollution
- Exposure to asbestos, uranium, chromium, arsenic, haematite

Histology

- Squamous carcinoma (50 per cent)
- Small-cell carcinoma (35 per cent)
- Adenocarcinoma (14 per cent)
- Others (<1 per cent)

Spread

- Direct to pleura, recurrent laryngeal nerve, pericardium, oesophagus, brachial plexus
- Lymphatic to mediastinal and cervical nodes
- Haematogenous to liver, bone, brain and adrenals
- Transcoelomic pleural seedlings and effusion

INVESTIGATIONS

- Chest X-ray: posteroanterior and lateral (lung opacity, hilar lymphadenopathy)

- Sputum cytology
- Bronchoscopy and cytology of brushings or lavage fluid
- CT-guided lung biopsy

MANAGEMENT

This depends on type, size, stage and spread.

Chemotherapy

- Indicated in small-cell carcinoma where initial response is often good
- Usually used for palliation in non small-cell carcinoma

Surgery

- Non small-cell tumours only
- Tumour confined to one lobe or lung
- No evidence of secondary deposits
- Good underlying performance status/lung function
- Operation: lobectomy or pneumonectomy
- Chemotherapy may be used in conjunction with surgery and radiotherapy

Palliative

- Radiotherapy (small-cell carcinoma most radiosensitive)
- May prevent haemoptysis, relieve bone pain from secondary deposits and relieve superior vena cava obstruction in all forms of bronchial carcinoma

PROGNOSIS

- Following 'curative' resection 5-year survival rates are approximately 20–30 per cent
- The overall 5-year survival is only about 6 per cent

CLUBBING

Fingernail clubbing is a key sign to discover on examination and an indication of several potentially life-threatening conditions.

Clubbing is defined as bulbous enlargement of the distal digits due to connective tissue proliferation.

FEATURES

- Loss of normal <165° 'Lovibond' angle between the nail and the cuticle (see Figure 2.4)
- Bogginess and fluctuation of the nail bed
- Increased curvature of the nail bed (all directions)
- Swelling of the distal digit, resembling drumsticks

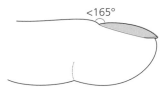

Figure 2.4 Lovibond angle

CAUSES

- Respiratory:
  - Bronchial carcinoma
  - Mesothelioma
  - Chronic suppurative lung diseases, e.g. cystic fibrosis, bronchiectasis
  - IPF
  - Empyema
- Cardiovascular:
  - Cyanotic heart disease (congenital)
  - Subacute bacterial endocarditis
  - Atrial myxoma
- Gastrointestinal:
  - Crohn's disease and ulcerative colitis
  - Cirrhosis
  - Coeliac disease
- Others:
  - Familial
  - Idiopathic
  - Thyroid acropachy (hyperthyroidism – resembles clubbing)

INVESTIGATING THE CAUSE

- Full history – including duration and family history for above diseases
- Full examination – for any signs suggestive of the above
- Investigations – baseline blood tests, urinalysis and imaging of the chest and abdomen may provide important clues

PLEURAL EFFUSION

DEFINITION

Pleural effusion is an abnormal accumulation of fluid between the visceral and parietal pleura of the lung.

HISTORY

- Asymptomatic (incidental finding)
- Shortness of breath
- Chest pain

- Concurrent upper respiratory tract infection
- known malignancy

EXAMINATION

Findings depend on severity of effusion:

- Increased respiratory rate
- Use accessory muscle
- Tracheal deviation
- Reduced chest expansion (on affected side)
- Stony dullness to percussion
- Reduced tactile vocal fremitus
- Reduced breath sounds
- Bronchial breathing above area of dullness

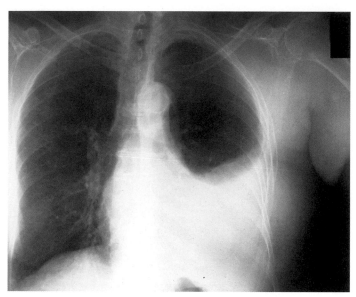

Figure 2.5 Radiograph showing pleural effusion (left)

INVESTIGATIONS

- Chest X-ray – uniform opacity, situated at the lung base on erect film
- Ultrasound scan – fluid directly imaged
- CT scan – fluid directly imaged
- Thoracocentesis – typical biochemical, cytological or microbiological profile (see Box 2.18)
- Pleural biopsy – histological diagnosis
- Thoracoscopy – direct visualization of the pleural space

BOX 2.18 THORACOCENTESIS RESULTS

Biochemistry:

- Protein: >30 g/dL exudate; <30 g/dL transudate
- LDH: >200 IU/mL exudate; <200 IU/mL transudate
- Glucose: low if less than half of serum glucose in rheumatoid arthritis, systemic lupus erythematosus, malignancy, tuberculosis and empyema
- pH: <7.1 in empyema
- Amylase: raised in pancreatitis
- Microscopy: white cell count, red blood cell count
- Cytology: malignant cells may be isolated

CAUSES

They can be subdivided according to whether the fluid is a transudate or an exudate, as follows:

- Transudate (<30 g/dL protein)
  - Nephrotic syndrome
  - Congestive cardiac failure
  - Cirrhosis
- Exudate (>30 g/dL protein)
  - Malignancy (primary or secondary)
  - Tuberculosis
  - Para-pneumonic
  - Rheumatoid arthritis, systemic lupus erythematosus
  - Pulmonary embolus

CYSTIC FIBROSIS

Cystic fibrosis is an autosomal recessive disease predominantly affecting Caucasians, with a heterozygote carrier rate of 1 in 20. Its clinical manifestations are due to an abnormality in chloride transport resulting in an excess of sodium and increase in viscosity of secretions.

HISTORY

General

- Symptoms often start in childhood
- Parents comment child tastes salty when they kiss them
- Failure to thrive

Respiratory

- Shortness of breath
- Cough with large volume sputum production
- Asthma poorly responsive to treatment
- Bronchiectasis
- Recurrent chest infections
- Sinusitis

Gastrointestinal

- Pancreatic failure
  - ○ Steatorrhoea and malabsorption
  - ○ Diabetes
- Diarrhoea/malabsorption
- Intussusception
- Gallstones
- Meconium ileus (newborns)

Infertility

- Males – obstruction or failure of development of vas deferens
- Females – subfertile due to irregular periods or abnormal mucus

EXAMINATION

General

- Young patient
- Pale
- Low body mass index (BMI), short stature

Respiratory

- Clubbing
- Short of breath
- Productive cough
- Added sounds:
  - ○ Inspiratory clicks
  - ○ Polyphonic expiratory wheeze
- Crepitations, especially over any areas of bronchiectasis

Gastrointestinal

- Rectal prolapse

INVESTIGATIONS

- Chest X-ray – tramlines of bronchiectasis
- CT scan thorax – widened, thickened bronchial walls
- Sodium sweat test (>60–70 mmol/L)
- Genetic analysis

COMPLICATIONS

- Recurrent upper respiratory tract infections
- Bronchiectasis
- Cor pulmonale
- Amyloidosis (secondary)
- Pancreatic insufficiency
- Abdominal pain and malabsorption
- Diabetes
- Infertility

TREATMENT

- Daily physiotherapy, percussion, postural drainage
- Prophylactic broad spectrum antibiotics (many will eventually become colonized with *Pseudomonas aeruginosa*)
- Bronchodilators
- Antimucolytic agents
- Immunization
- Pancreatic enzyme replacement
- Lung transplantation in selected cases

BRONCHIECTASIS

This respiratory disease manifests itself as a result of several disease processes. It results in dilatation of the large airways, significant sputum production and recurrent respiratory tract infections.

HISTORY

- Shortness of breath
- Cough with large volume sputum production
- Wheeze
- Cystic fibrosis

EXAMINATION

- Full sputum pot next to bed
- Clubbing
- Short of breath
- Productive cough
- Added sounds:
  - Inspiratory clicks
  - Polyphonic expiratory wheeze
- Crepitations especially over any areas of bronchiectasis
- Respiratory failure, e.g. cyanosis
- Cor pulmonale

BOX 2.19 CAUSES OF BRONCHIECTASIS

- Cystic fibrosis
- Secondary to chronic infection (e.g. tuberculosis, pneumonia)
- Primary ciliary dyskinesis (Kartagener's syndrome)
- Hypogammaglobulinaemia
- Allergic bronchopulmonary aspergillosis
- Endobronchial obstruction

INVESTIGATIONS

- Chest X-ray – tramlines (bronchial wall thickening)
- CT scan thorax

COMPLICATIONS

- Secondary amyloidosis
- Empyema
- Right heart failure (cor pulmonale)

ABDOMEN

ABDOMINAL EXAMINATION

INTRODUCTION

- Introduce yourself, explain procedure and request permission
- Enquire about any pain or discomfort
- Ensure adequate lighting
- Expose the patient appropriately – ideally from 'nipples to knees'
- Lie flat

INSPECTION

General

- Cachexia, jaundice, pigmentation scars
- Distension, ascites
- Spider naevi, distended veins, caput medusae
- Tattoos, track marks

Hands

- Clubbing, anaemia
- Koilonychia, leukonychia
- Palmar erythema, Dupuytren's contracture
- Liver flap
- Tendon xanthoma

Eyes

- Anaemia
- Jaundice
- Xanthelasma (e.g. primary biliary cirrhosis)

Mouth

- Angular stomatitis, mouth ulcers (inflammatory bowel disease)
- Candida, tongue dryness, smoothness
- Brown macules on lips, periorally and buccal mucosa e.g. Peutz–Jeghers disease – associated with hamartomatous gut polyps that are prone to bleeding, malignancy
- Telangiectasia on tongue, periorally and lips, e.g. Osler–Weber–Rendu syndrome – also gastrointestinal telangiectasia that can bleed

Neck
- Lymphadenopathy – particularly left supraclavicular (Virchow's node, metastatic invasion seen in visceral cancer – Troisier's sign)
- Jugular venous pressure – may be raised in liver disease caused by right-sided heart failure

Abdomen

As above:

- Caput medusae, striae, ascites
- Visible pulsation or peristalsis
- Hernias or scars

PALPATION

Kneel down, with the patient lying flat while observing the patient's face. Palpate lightly then deep, over the four quadrants (right and left upper, right and left lower; see Figure 1.2, p. 9). Start farthest from any tender point.

Palpate for any:

- Guarding
- Tenderness and rebound tenderness on releasing pressure
- Masses
- Organomegaly
- Ascites

BOX 2.20 DIFFERENTIAL DIAGNOSIS OF ABDOMINAL DISTENSION

5 Fs:
- Fat
- Flatus
- Faeces
- Fetus
- Fluid

BOX 2.21 ORGAN-SPECIFIC CAUSES OF ABDOMINAL MASSES

- Hepatomegaly
- Gall bladder enlargement (e.g. cancer, empyema)
- Splenomegaly (infection, lymphoproliferative disease)
- Bowel (cancer, obstruction, faeces, Crohn's mass)
- Pancreas (cysts, cancer)
- Stomach (pyloric stenosis, distension, cancer)
- Kidneys (polycystic, hydronephrosis, cancer)
- Aorta (aneurysm)
- Uterus (pregnancy, cancer, fibroids)
- Ovary/fallopian tubes (cysts, cancer, ectopic pregnancy)
- Bladder (retention, cancer)
- Others – hernia, lipoma, lymphadenopathy, ascites

Organomegaly

- Liver:
  - Feel sequentially with radial edge of hand on deep inspiration, starting in right iliac fossa (RIF) moving towards right upper quadrant (RUQ)
  - Note size of hepatomegaly in finger breadths or centimetres
  - Note character: smooth, craggy, tender
- Spleen:
  - Feel sequentially with radial edge of hand on deep inspiration, starting in RIF moving diagonally towards left upper quadrant (LUQ)
  - Note size of splenomegaly
  - Note character and presence/absence of notch
  - Note nature of percussion note over spleen and whether you can get above it (see Box 2.22)
- Kidneys:
  - Feel bilaterally for loin masses or tenderness
  - Ballot bimanually
  - Note size, surface and overlying percussion note

BOX 2.22 DIFFERENTIATING BETWEEN SPLENOMEGALY OR ENLARGED KIDNEY

Spleen:
- Cannot get above it
- Overlying percussion note is dull
- Moves down and out on respiration
- Palpable notch on medial side

Kidney:
- Can get above it
- Resonant percussion note
- Will not move on respiration
- No notch palpable

Abdominal aortic aneurysm (see p. 68)

- Palpate with two hands roughly 3 cm lateral (left) and superior to the umbilicus
- Note the character of the aortic pulse – aneurysms are expansile, pulsatile masses

PERCUSSION

- Liver and spleen in directions outlined above
- Masses
- Bladder
- Ascites (shifting dullness and fluid thrill)

AUSCULTATION

- Listen for:
  - Presence/absence or abnormal 'tinkling' bowel sounds
  - Bruits over kidneys, aorta, liver
  - Rubs (liver/splenic)

COMPLETE EXAMINATION

- Offer to:
  - Examine hernial orifices
  - Examine external genitalia
  - Perform a rectal examination (see p. 61)

BOX 2.23 PALPATING FOR ASCITES

Shifting dullness:
- Percuss into the flanks bilaterally
- Note an area where it changes from resonant to dull, on the left side
- Keep hand in position and ask patient to roll towards you and wait for a minute
- The percussion note should now be resonant throughout this side if there is ascites, due to fluid movement

Fluid thrill:
- If the abdomen is tense with ascites ask the patient to place the ulnar border of their hand over the umbilicus, down the centre of the abdomen
- Place your left hand on the left abdominal ward and 'flick' the skin of the right side
- A fluid thrill should be felt in tense ascites by the left hand

---

INVESTIGATIONS

- Dipstick urine
- Full set of blood tests (depending on findings)
- Imaging e.g. ultrasound or CT scan.

RECTAL EXAMINATION

INTRODUCTION

- Explain the examination: may be uncomfortable but to alert you if painful
- Request permission
- Arrange for a chaperone
- Ensure doors are locked and curtains drawn around patient to prevent interruption
- Position patient lying in the left lateral position with the buttocks on edge of bed and knees raised to the chest
- Expose appropriately
- Put gloves on and obtain some aqueous jelly

INSPECTION

Look for:

- Inflammation
- Lesions
  - Skin tags
  - External haemorrhoids (extend into canal)
  - Perianal haematoma (localized to verge alone)
  - Perianal warts
  - Fissures (spread anal verge to flatten rugae – commonest posteriorly)

EXAMINATION

- Warn patient that you are starting internal examination
- Lubricate gloved index finger

- Insert through rectum with pulp of finger pointing posteriorly
- Palpate posterior wall
- Rotate finger to examine anteriorly for:
  - Prostate in males: note size, shape and consistency
    - Normal: walnut size, smooth
    - Malignant: craggy, enlarged
    - Benign prostatic hypertrophy: enlarged, smooth
  - Vagina in females
    - Examine lateral walls for tenderness: may suggest abscess/inflammation
  - Right side – appendicitis
  - Left side – diverticulitis
- Any masses: surface, consistency, position (note according to a clock face)
- Examine faecal material on glove
  - Colour e.g. black: melaena
  - Blood – altered/fresh
  - Mucus
- Clean anus with gauze at the end of the examination

Note:

- Haemorrhoids are *not* palpable unless thrombosed
- Internal haemorrhoids can only be assessed using proctoscope

TESTICULAR EXAMINATION

INTRODUCTION

- Explain the examination
- Ask if there is any pain
- Request permission and invite a chaperone
- Position patient standing
- Expose umbilicus to knees
- Consider wearing gloves

INSPECTION

- Ensure you examine anterior and posterior aspects of scrotum
- Lumps or swellings – inguinal or scrotal
- Skin:
  - Scars
  - Colour/temperature, e.g. erythematous, hot
  - Ulcers, e.g. herpetic – clusters of vesicles, painless
  - Carcinoma – indurated, friable

PALPATION

- Testes:
  - Roll testes gently between your thumb and index finger
    - Ensure both palpable and roughly equal
    - Assess any masses: see Box 2.24

- Epididymis (above and posterior to testis):
  - ○ Swelling
  - ○ Masses
- Feel along spermatic cord

BOX 2.24 ASSESSING SCROTAL LUMPS

- Size
- Shape
- Surface
- Consistency
- Fluctuance
- Transillumination: shine light from behind mass
- Tenderness (torsion, epididymo-orchitis)

AUSCULTATION

Bowel sounds may be heard in a grossly distended sac of an indirect inguinal hernia containing abdominal contents.

TRANSILLUMINATION

Fluid-containing testicular swellings such as hydroceles can be illuminated with a torch.

BOX 2.25 TESTICULAR SWELLINGS

Painless swellings:
- Testicular tumour – attached to testis, irregular, craggy and hard, may have secondary hydrocele
- Hydrocele – diffuse, fluctuant, transilluminable, can get above it, cannot feel it discretely from testicle
- Indirect hernia – cannot get above it, felt separately to testis, may contain bowel
- Epididymal cyst – felt separate to and above testis, attached to epididymis, e.g. spermatocoele
- Varicocele – dilation of venous plexus, 'bag of worms' felt on standing, separate to testis, often on left

Painful swellings:
- Testicular torsion – acutely tender, swollen, elevated testicle – note: surgical emergency
- Epididymo-orchitis – tender, swollen epididymis ± testicular swelling

---

COMPLETE EXAMINATION

Offer to examine:

- The abdomen
- The external genitalia
- Per rectum

INVESTIGATIONS

- Urinalysis
- Urethral swabs
- Depending on findings consider formal genitourinary medicine or urology referral

LYMPHADENOPATHY

INTRODUCTION

- Explain the examination
- Ask about painful areas/lumps
- Request permission
- Position patient sitting up
- Expose appropriately: underwear only – but cover patient appropriately while examining upper body

INSPECTION

- Lumps or swellings (ask the patient to point out any lumps)
- Skin changes – rash, erythema
- Scars or scratch marks
- Bruising or purpura
- Cachexia
- Joint deformities

PALPATION

Ask if there is any tenderness in each region.

Head and neck

- Examine from behind the patient using fingertips
- Under chin (submental) moving to angle of jaw (submandibular)
- Move up jaw to in front (preauricular) and behind ear (postauricular)
- Move thumbs to back of head to palpate occipital nodes
- Then along anterior border of sternocleidomastoid to palpate cervical nodes that run along internal jugular vein
- Then move onto supraclavicular fossa paying particular attention to Virchow's node (angle of sternocleidomastoid and clavicle) – suggests intra-abdominal malignancy

Axilla (five regions)

- Turn patient facing you
- Take left hand in your left hand to examine right axilla and vice versa
- Ensure patient arm is relaxed – 'let me take all the weight of your arm'
- Palpate each region in turn – anterior, posterior, lateral, medial and apical

Groin – superficial inguinal nodes

- Expose groin to knee

- Palpate the anterior superior iliac spine (ASIS) and pubic tubercle to delineate the inguinal ligament
- Palpate just below the ligament
- Then move along just medial to sartorius to palpate subinguinal nodes

---

BOX 2.26 DIFFERENTIAL DIAGNOSIS OF LYMPHADENOPATHY

Infection
- Bacterial, e.g. tuberculosis, *Streptococcus*, syphilis
- Viral, e.g. mumps, Epstein–Barr virus, human immunodeficiency virus (HIV)
- Others, e.g. toxoplasmosis

Autoimmune
- Sarcoidosis
- Systemic lupus erythematosus

Malignancy
- Primary: lymphomas, leukaemias
- Secondary: spread from e.g. stomach, ovary

FURTHER EXAMINATION

Offer to examine:

- The area draining to the involved node:
  - Cervical:
    - Head and neck
    - Oral cavity
    - Larynx
    - Pharynx
  - Axilla:
    - Arm
    - Breast
    - Abdomen/chest wall above umbilicus
  - Inguinal:
    - Leg
    - Buttock
    - Perineum (scrotum/anal canal)
    - Abdominal wall below umbilicus

  Note: Testes drain to para-aortic lymph nodes along course of gonadal vessels not to the inguinal nodes
- The abdomen, e.g. for hepato/splenomegaly

BOX 2.27 EXAMINING LUMPS

- Site: which group of nodes
- Size: larger than 1 cm is significant
- Shape
- Surface/edges: smooth versus irregular
- Consistency: hard suggestive of neoplastic process
- Fixation: suggests local malignant infiltration
- Temperature: warm likely reactive/infective
- Tenderness: more likely infective
- Overlying skin: tethering in carcinomas, erythema in infection

HERNIAS

INTRODUCTION

- Explain the examination
- Ask about painful areas
- Request permission
- Position patient lying flat with arms by their sides and head rested
- Expose appropriately – 'nipples to knees'

INSPECTION

- Scars (an incisional hernia may arise from any scar)
- Old inguinal incisions (recurrence, contralateral hernia)
- If no obvious swellings while lying, ask patient to stand
- Observe from front and side
- Note position in relation to pubic tubercle and extension into the scrotum on deep ring (midway between the ASIS and pubic tubercle)

BOX 2.28 TYPES OF GROIN HERNIAS

Inguinal: neck superior and medial to pubic tubercle
- **Direct** – reduce directly backwards, appear medial to deep ring therefore not controlled by pressure over it, do not extend into scrotum
- **Indirect** – reduce up and laterally, controlled by pressure over deep ring, may extend into scrotum (most common type of hernia overall)

Femoral: neck inferior and lateral to pubic tubercle, small, firm, may not feel cough impulse (more common in women)

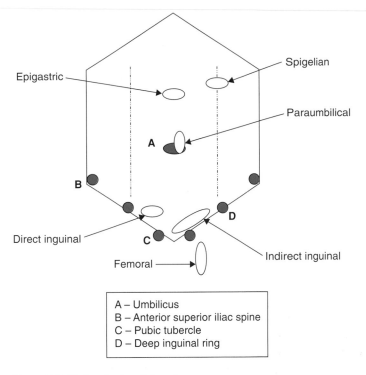

Figure 2.6 Abdominal wall hernias

PALPATION

If still no swelling on standing ask patient to cough each time while palpating as follows:

- Epigastrium: hand flat on abdomen with wrist above umbilicus and fingers extending to sternum
- Umbilicus: with fingertips over umbilicus
- Palpate any scars
- Groin: hand pressed obliquely with wrist over the ASIS and fingertips extending to pubic tubercle
- Note: Even if obvious hernia located continue to examine all sites – there may be more than one.

ASSESS

- Position – in relation to pubic tubercle/ASIS
- Extension into the scrotum (indirect hernia)
- Temperature
- Tenderness
- Size
- Tension
- Cough impulse: compress firmly and ask patient to turn away and cough – feel bulging onto your fingers
- Reducibility

AUSCULTATION

- Bowel sounds may be present

TRANSILLUMINATION

- Ascites/hydrocele/cystic fluid

COMPLETE EXAMINATION

- Examine both sides
- Offer to examine:
  - Rest of abdomen
  - External genitalia
  - Per rectum

BOX 2.29 COMPLICATIONS OF GROIN HERNIAS

- **Incarceration** – soft, will need surgery to prevent bowel injury
- **Strangulation** – irreducible, tender, tense, no cough impulse, may have systemic upset, needs surgery as an emergency

---

ABDOMINAL AORTIC ANEURYSM

An abdominal aortic aneurysm (AAA) is a localized dilatation of the abdominal aorta, that exceeds the normal diameter by more than 50 per cent (normal diameter = 2 cm, therefore rule of thumb: >3 cm abnormal).

AETIOLOGY

Essentially unknown. Potential theories:

- Genetic
- Atherosclerosis
- Infection
- Connective tissue disorders (Marfan's)
- Trauma

Facts:

- 90 per cent are infrarenal
- Male to female ratio – 5:1
- Peak age 80 years

RISK FACTORS

- Family history: 25 per cent have first-degree relative
- Previous aneurysm repair
- Peripheral aneurysm (popliteal or femoral)
- Smoking (prevalence increases ×8)

- Coronary artery disease
- Hypertension

PRESENTATION

- Asymptomatic:
  - Incidental finding usually on ultrasound scan
  - Palpable pulsatile expansive mass
- Rupture:
  - Classic triad: hypotension, back pain, pulsatile abdominal mass
  - Grey–Turner sign (flank bruising indicates retroperitoneal haemorrhage)
  - 90 per cent mortality, 50 per cent if survive to the operating theatre
- Peripheral embolus:
  - Ischaemic foot/digits
  - Livedo reticularis of the feet or blue toe syndrome
- Acute occlusion – acute claudication, usually bilaterally to the buttocks (indicates high occlusion)
- Fistulation:
  - Aortocaval: tachycardia, congestive cardiac failure, abdominal thrill/bruit, renal failure, and peripheral ischemia
  - Aortoduodenal: into fourth part of duodenum: herald upper gastrointestinal bleed followed by an often fatal exsanguinating haemorrhage

MANAGEMENT

- <5 cm: surveillance with 6-monthly ultrasound scans. Operate if become symptomatic or rapidly increase in size
- >5 cm risk of rupture increases exponentially. Operate but must consider operative risk. If very high risk there is a role for monitoring and surveillance
- In women rupture risk is higher at smaller diameters, therefore consider operating at >4 cm
- Screening with abdominal ultrasonography is now being considered for all men aged 65 years and over

SURGERY

- Traditional open repair
- Minimally invasive endovascular repair

COMPLICATIONS

- Death (up to 5 per cent in elective, 50 per cent in emergency)
- Pneumonia, myocardial infarction, renal failure
- Wound infection
- Graft infection
- Incisional hernia
- Emboli, distal ischaemia, blue toe syndrome
- Impotence in men
- Late graft enteric fistula (any gastrointestinal bleed at any time post-AAA repair needs full investigation. Initial bleed may herald total exsanguination)

CHRONIC LIVER DISEASE

Chronic liver disease is a common disease frequently encountered in the OSCE and essentially comprises many of the features you would inspect for in an abdominal examination.

INSPECTION
General

- Weight loss, jaundice/pigmentation and scars
- Abdominal distension, ascites
- Spider naevi, distended veins, caput medusae
- Tattoos, track marks
- Gynaecomastia

BOX 2.30 CAUSES OF CHRONIC LIVER DISEASE

Infective:
- Bacterial, e.g. leptospirosis
- Viral, e.g. hepatitis B and C
- Parasitic, e.g. schistosomiasis, malaria

Metabolic:
- Wilson's disease
- Haemochromatosis
- α-antitrypsin deficiency

Malignant:
- Primary: hepatocellular carcinoma
- Secondary: metastases

Drugs:
- Alcohol
- Paracetamol
- Statins
- Vitamin A derivatives

Others:
- Chronic active hepatitis
- CCF
- Primary biliary cirrhosis

Hands

- Clubbing, anaemia
- Koilonychia, leukonychia
- Palmar erythema, Dupuytren's contracture
- Asterixis (liver flap)
- Tendon xanthoma

Eyes

- Anaemia
- Jaundice
- Xanthelasma (e.g. primary biliary cirrhosis)

Neck

- Lymphadenopathy – particularly left supraclavicular (Virchow's node, metastatic invasion seen in visceral cancer – Troisier's sign)
- Jugular venous pressure – may be raised

PALPATION

- Hepatomegaly ± splenomegaly
- Bilateral enlarged kidneys (polycystic kidney disease [PCKD] can affect the liver too)

AUSCULTATE

- Bruits over the liver (hepatoma)
- Rubs (liver/splenic)

INVESTIGATIONS

- Liver screen – see Box 2.31
- Ultrasound scan abdomen
- CT scan abdomen and pelvis

BOX 2.31 LIVER SCREEN BLOOD TESTS

- Haematology – coagulation
- Biochemistry – liver function tests, γ-glutamyl transferase, aspartate transaminase, copper and caeruloplasmin, iron studies, ferritin, α_1-antitrypsin
- Immunology – antinuclear antibodies, antimitochondrial antibodies, anti-smooth muscle antibodies, anti-LKM1 antibodies and tissue transglutaminase antibodies
- Microbiology – hepatitis A, B and C, cytomegalovirus, Epstein–Barr virus

---

COMPLICATIONS

- Immunosuppression
- Portal hypertension – oesophageal varices
- Clotting derangement
- Cirrhosis
- Wernicke's encephalopathy and Korsakoff's Psychosis

CHRONIC KIDNEY DISEASE AND RENAL TRANSPLANTS

Renal patients, with or without transplants, are commonly encountered in finals examinations as they provide a wealth of physical signs.

BOX 2.32 CAUSES OF RENAL FAILURE

- Pre-renal, e.g. hypovolaemia, sepsis
- Renal, e.g. vascular disease, glomerular disease
- Post-renal, i.e. obstructive, e.g. prostatic hypertrophy, urethral stricture, retroperitoneal fibrosis

---

INSPECTION

General

- Scars from:
  - Previous central lines (neck), subclavian lines
  - Peritoneal dialysis catheters
  - Renal transplants
  - Nephrectomy
  - Insulin injection sites
- Arteriovenous fistulae on forearms
- Joint disease due to hyperparathyroidism
- Uraemic 'frost'

Face

- Hearing aid – suggesting cause for renal failure, e.g. Alport's
- Lipodystrophy – rarely seen in some forms of glomerulonephritis
- Parathyroidectomy scar – from tertiary hyperparathyroidism
- Cushingoid ('moon') face – from steroid therapy
- Gum hypertrophy – from ciclosporin therapy
- Hirsutism – ciclosporin

Abdomen

- Scars (see above)
- Lipodystrophy from insulin injection (i.e. diabetes)
- Swelling (and scar) from renal transplant

BOX 2.33 COMMON CAUSES OF RENAL FAILURE REQUIRING TRANSPLANT

- Hypertension
- Diabetes mellitus
- Glomerulonephritis
- Chronic pyelonephritis
- PCKD

EXAMINATION

- Signs of anaemia – conjunctival pallor
- Assessment of fluid balance:
  - JVP
  - Blood pressure

- ○ Peripheral oedema
- ○ Pleural effusions
- ○ Daily weight
- Arteriovenous fistula – buzzing or not, bruit heard over it
- Pericarditis – pericardial rub
- Abdomen:
  - ○ Enlarged ballottable loin masses
    - ◆ Polycystic kidneys
    - ◆ Hydronephrosis
  - ○ Palpable mass in right (or left) iliac fossa with overlying scar – transplanted kidney
  - ○ Enlarged liver, e.g. polycystic liver
- Nervous system – the following are all suggestive of uraemia:
  - ○ Reduced consciousness/confusion
  - ○ Peripheral neuropathy
  - ○ Myoclonus

INVESTIGATIONS

- Urea and electrolytes
- FBC, liver function tests (LFTs), bone profile, ESR, creatine kinase (CK) and clotting screen
- Autoimmune screen, e.g. antinuclear antibody, antineutrophilic cytoplasmic antibodies, dsDNA, complement
- Virology, e.g. hepatitis, HIV
- Urinalysis and microscopy
- ECG
- Chest X-ray
- Renal tract ultrasound scan
- If polycystic disease confirmed, associated cerebral berry aneurysm formation can be detected with magnetic resonance imaging (MRI)

BOX 2.34 COMMON BLOOD TEST RESULTS IN RENAL FAILURE

- FBC: normocytic, normochromic anaemia, thrombocytopenia
- Urea and creatinine: raised
- Potassium: raised (if severe)
- Calcium: hypocalcaemia, rarely hypercalcaemia if tertiary hyperparathyroidism develops
- Phosphate: hyperphosphataemia
- High parathyroid hormone levels
- Acid–base balance: low bicarbonate
- Dyslipidaemia

MANAGEMENT

- Treat the underlying disease process
- Treat associated diseases, e.g. coronary artery disease

- Avoid nephrotoxic medications, e.g. contrast, aminoglycosides
- Tight control of blood pressure
- Statin or other hyperlipidaemia medication
- ACE inhibitors/angiotensin II blockers
- Erythropoietin for anaemia
- Calcium + calcitriol, phosphate binders
- Dialysis: haemodialysis or peritoneal
- Transplantation

ADULT POLYCYSTIC KIDNEY DISEASE

Adult PCKD is an inherited autosomal disorder that commonly presents in mid-adulthood. Cysts may occur in the kidneys, liver, pancreas and ovaries.

HISTORY

- Loin pain
- Haematuria
- Urinary tract infection
- Renal failure

EXAMINATION

- Loin masses
- Enlarged irregular liver (also polycystic)
- Hypertension
- Anaemia (secondary to renal failure)
- Evidence of renal failure (see p. 71):
  - Arteriovenous (AV) fistulae
  - Continuous ambulatory peritoneal dialysis (CAPD) scars
  - Nephrectomy scar
  - Renal transplant

COMPLICATIONS

- Chronic renal failure
- Cyst infection or bleeding (causing pain)
- Cerebral (berry) aneurysm and rupture
- Mitral valve prolapse
- Renal stones

INVESTIGATIONS

- Gene analysis
- Ultrasound scan

MYELOPROLIFERATIVE AND LYMPHOPROLIFERATIVE DISEASES

This topic incorporates a wide range of diseases that presents with similar signs such as hepatosplenomegaly that are not uncommon in final clinical examinations.

HISTORY

- Weight loss
- Fever
- Night sweats
- Itching
- Symptoms and signs of an abnormal blood count:
  - Low platelets: easy bruising, bleeding, e.g. epistaxis
  - Neutropenia: infection
  - Anaemia: lethargy, malaise, shortness of breath, chest pain, pallor
- Painful, distended abdomen and/or lymph nodes
- Myalgia

BOX 2.35 MYELOPROLIFERATIVE AND LYMPHOPROLIFERATIVE DISEASES

- Acute myeloid leukaemia: younger population, rapid onset
- Chronic myeloid leukaemia (CML): older men, raised white cell count, splenomegaly, Philadelphia chromosome common
- Acute lymphoblastic leukaemia: commonly occurs in children
- Chronic lymphocytic leukaemia (CLL): mostly adults >60 years, two-thirds are men
- Multiple myeloma: older adults, multiple bony lesions
- Myelodysplastic disease (MDS): adults, ineffective blood cell production
- Myelofibrosis: older adults, bone marrow fibrosis
- Hodgkin's lymphoma: bimodal peaks in young and older adults
- Non-Hodgkin's lymphoma: more common in adults

EXAMINATION

- Anaemia: pale conjunctivae
- Petechiae (owing to low platelets)
- Infections (owing to immunosuppression), e.g. herpes zoster, oral thrush
- Lymphadenopathy – nodes may be 'rubbery' in texture (see p. 64)
- Splenomegaly – may be massive (arises from left upper quadrant and extending to right iliac fossa, notched edge, unable to get above it)
- Hepatomegaly

BOX 2.36 CAUSES OF SPLENOMEGALY

- Lymphoproliferative diseases: CLL, lymphoma
- Myeloproliferative diseases: CML, myelofibrosis
- Infections: bacterial endocarditis, hepatitis, leishmaniasis, malaria
- Inflammatory: sarcoidosis, Felty's syndrome, systemic lupus erythematosus
- Infiltration: amyloidosis, Gaucher's syndrome
- Congestion: hepatic vein thrombosis, portal hypertension, congestive cardiac failure

---

INVESTIGATIONS

- FBC
- Peripheral blood film
- Cytogenetic analysis, e.g. for Philadelphia translocation
- Imaging, e.g. ultrasound scan abdomen, CT scan, positron emission tomography (PET) scan
- Lymph node/bone marrow biopsy
- Lumbar puncture (for central nervous system [CNS] involvement and treatment)

TREATMENT

(Depending on diagnosis)

- Multidisciplinary team approach, i.e. including specialist nurses, physiotherapy, pharmacist, psychologist, etc.
- Chemotherapy
- Tyrosine kinase inhibitors
- Bone marrow transplant

NEUROLOGY

PERIPHERAL NERVOUS SYSTEM EXAMINATION

INTRODUCTION

- Introduce yourself, explain procedure and request permission
- Enquire about any pain or discomfort
- Ensure adequate lighting
- Position patient on a couch with arms and legs exposed

EXAMINATION

Inspection:	Is
Tone:	This
Power:	Physician
Reflexes:	Really
Sensation:	So
Coordination:	Cool?

INSPECTION

- Asymmetry
- Swelling
- Scars
- Deformity
- Wasting or hypertrophy
- Fasciculation
- Abnormal movements or posturing
- Hypomimia

Upper limb

Ask patient to hold arms out straight in front of them with palms facing the ceiling. Look for:

- Tremor (resting, intention, coarse, fine, frequency)
- Pronator drift when eyes closed – corresponds to upper motor neurone (UMN) lesion
- Rebound (overshoot seen in cerebellar disease)

TONE

Assess tone by moving joints slowly and quickly at:

- Wrist/elbow/shoulder
- Ankle/knee

BOX 2.37 COMMON TONE ABNORMALITIES

- Hypertonic/spastic, e.g. after central lesion
- Clasp knife (increased tone and sudden release) – pyramidal tract lesion
- Lead-pipe, uniform rigidity – Parkinson's
- Cog-wheeling – tremor superimposed on rigidity at wrist in Parkinson's
- Hypotonia – lower motor neurone (LMN lesions), recent UMN and cerebellar lesions

---

POWER

Compare left with right by applying resistance to movements of:

- Upper limb:
  - Push arms up and down 'like wings'
  - Hold left elbow in left hand, and forearm in right and assess biceps flexion and triceps extension power with right hand. Repeat in other arm
  - Arms out straight – assess wrist extension and flexion with same hand bilaterally
  - Squeeze two of your fingers in the patient's fist as tight as possible (intrinsic muscles C8–T1)
  - Spread fingers apart – keep apart and compare 'like with like', i.e. first finger against first and little finger against little (C7)
  - Hold piece of paper between middle and ring fingers and pull (interossei, ulnar nerve)
  - Assess pincer grip against own (opponens pollicis, median nerve)
  - Assess thumb abduction – 'push thumbs to the ceiling' (median nerve)
- Lower limb
  - Straight leg raise (push down on thigh) and push leg down onto bed (hand under thigh)
  - Bend knees up. In turn extend the knees against resistance ('kick away' legs) and then flex knees ('pull heels to your bottom')
  - Lie legs flat and assess ankle flexion and extension, in turn
  - Assess big toe flexion and extension (normally very strong)

BOX 2.38 CAUSES OF REDUCED POWER

UMN
- Cerebrovascular disease
- Space occupying lesion
- Multiple sclerosis
- Spinal injury

LMN
- Peripheral neuropathy, e.g. B vitamin deficiencies
- Motor neurone disease
- Radiculopathy
- Polio
- Guillain–Barré syndrome

MYOPATHY
- Disuse
- Muscular dystrophy
- Alcohol

REFLEXES
- Hold the tendon hammer near its end and let it 'fall' on the tendon in question, giving it a large trajectory
- Reinforce any absent or reduced reflexes with Jendrassik's manoeuvre (clench teeth, or pull apart interlocked finger tips and release before striking tendon)

Upper limb
- Biceps tendon – C5, 6
- Triceps tendon – C7, 8
- Supinator – C5, 6
- Finger reflexes

Lower limb
- Knee jerk – L3, 4
- Ankle jerk – S1, 2
- Plantar reflex

SENSATION
- Assess all dermatomes, demonstrating first on the sternum with eyes closed for:
  - Pin-prick
  - Light touch
  - Two-point discrimination
  - Temperature
- Vibration sense:
  - Assess at bony landmarks
  - Use 128 Hz tuning fork

BOX 2.39 DIFFERENTIATING UPPER AND LOWER MOTOR NEURONE PRESENTATIONS

UMN
- **I:** flexed arm, extended leg
- **T:** increased
- **P:** generally weak although flexors > extensors in upper limbs and extensors > flexors in lower limbs
- **R:** brisk
- **S:** abnormal, reduced, absent in affected limbs
- **C:** reduced

LMN
- **I:** wasting, fasciculation
- **T:** reduced
- **P:** generally weak
- **R:** reduced, absent
- **S:** reduced, abnormal
- **C:** impaired

- ○ Ask the patient to close their eyes and say yes when they feel the vibration similar to that demonstrated first on the sternum
  - ○ Progress superiorly until positive response elicited
  - ○ Start at big toe interphalangeal joint, then medial malleolus, knee, ASIS
- Proprioception
  - ○ Hold a joint e.g. the big toe interphalangeal joint at the sides
  - ○ Demonstrate to the patient upwards and downwards movement
  - ○ Ask them to then close their eyes and tell you in which direction you are moving the toe, making small adjustments up or down
  - ○ If unable to identify direction of movements accurately, move to proximal joints, e.g. ankle, knee, hip until intact

COORDINATION

- Upper limb:
  - ○ Ask the patient to touch your finger with their outstretched finger and then their nose
  - ○ Repeat
  - ○ May elicit intention tremor, poor coordination and past pointing
  - ○ Ask the patient to tap one hand on the other, alternating between the palmar and dorsal sides of the moving hand (dysdiadochokinesis). Repeat with the other hand
- Lower limb:
  - ○ Ask the patient to run their heel down the front of the shin, lift off the leg and return it to the knee and repeat the process
  - ○ Replicate in the contralateral leg

GAIT

- Assess the patient's gait, e.g. ataxic, antalgic, festinating
- Assess Romberg's sign (assesses dorsal columns and joint position sense)
  - Ask patient to stand with their feet together, hands by their sides and eyes open (note: be ready to help stabilize them if they appear as if they may fall!)
  - Then ask them to close their eyes
- Test is positive if patient sways or falls with eyes closed

FURTHER TESTS

- Bloods tests:
  - FBC, e.g. macrocytic anaemia – vitamin B_{12} deficiency, polycythaemia – stroke, raised white cell count – infection
  - Biochemistry, e.g. electrolyte disturbances, vitamin deficiencies
  - Thyroid function, e.g. hypothyroidism
  - Venereal disease research laboratory (VDRL) test – syphilis
  - *Borrelia* serology – Lyme disease
  - Autoantibody screen, e.g. systemic lupus erythematosus, Wegener's
- Lumbar puncture (see p. 229)
  - Protein: raised in multiple sclerosis (MS) and Guillain–Barré
  - Cell count: raised white cell count with meningitis, raised red blood cell count/xanthochromia in subarachnoid haemorrhage
  - Microscopy
- Electroencephalography: epileptiform activity
- Nerve conduction studies: peripheral neuropathy
- Electromyography: myopathy, myositis
- Imaging:
  - CT, e.g. to examine for space-occupying lesions, strokes
  - MRI brain, e.g. to examine for the above and multiple sclerosis

PERIPHERAL NEUROPATHY

There are myriad causes of peripheral neuropathy, often presenting with similar symptoms and signs.

HISTORY

- Limbs:
  - Muscle wasting
  - Narrowing of lower leg ('inverted champagne bottle' – HSMN)
  - Deformity: clawing of toes, pes cavus
  - Weakness
  - Foot-drop
  - Paraesthesia, dysaesthesia, hyperalgesia
  - Pain: burning, electric shock-like
  - Poor coordination

BOX 2.40 CAUSES OF PERIPHERAL NEUROPATHY

- Idiopathic: 10–20 per cent of cases
- Hereditary: hereditary sensory and motor neuropathy (HSMN 1 and 2)
- Drugs: alcohol, phenytoin, amiodarone, gold, ethambutol
- Toxins: lead, heavy metals, arsenic, solvents, insecticides
- Metabolic: diabetes mellitus, renal, liver and thyroid disease
- Vitamin deficiencies: A, B_1(thiamine), B_{12}, E
- Connective tissue: rheumatoid arthritis, systemic lupus erythematosus, vasculitides
- Malignancy: carcinomatous infiltration, chemotherapy agents
- Haematological: myeloma, monoclonal gammopathy of unknown significance (MGUS)
- Infections: HIV, syphilis, leprosy
- Others: sarcoidosis, amyloidosis, trauma and compression, Guillain–Barré syndrome

---

- ○ Tremor
- ○ Fasciculation
- ○ Autonomic dysfunction
- Gait:
  - ○ Ataxia, difficulty walking
  - ○ Falls
  - ○ Loss of balance
  - ○ High-stepping
  - ○ Foot drag
- Face:
  - ○ Facial muscle weakness: unilateral or bilateral, effective all muscle groups including the forehead
  - ○ Sensory abnormalities (see limbs above)
  - ○ Bulbar involvement, i.e. poor swallow
  - ○ Abnormal speech (see p. 95)

EXAMINATION

- Inspection (as above):
  - ○ Wasting
  - ○ Deformity
  - ○ Fasciculations
  - ○ Tremor
- Tone:
  - ○ Reduced – 'flaccid'
- Power:
  - ○ Reduced due to weakness if motor fibres are affected
- Reflexes:
  - ○ Diminished or absent
  - ○ Down-going plantars
- Sensation:
  - ○ Abnormal to complete loss

- ○ Absent proprioception and vibration sense may indicate dorsal column involvement (from vitamin B_{12} deficiency and subacute combined degeneration of the cord [SACD])
- Coordination
  - ○ Impaired

INVESTIGATIONS

- Identical to those for the peripheral nervous system (see p. 80)
- Nerve conduction studies: help differentiate between axonal and demyelinating disease

TREATMENT

- Treat underlying causes – stop alcohol, immunosuppress connective tissue disease, control diabetes. Not all neuropathies will improve
- Refer to chronic pain specialist
- Physiotherapy, orthotics and foot care

GAIT AND BALANCE

INTRODUCTION

- Introduce yourself to the patient
- Explain the examination and gain consent
- Confirm that the patient is able to walk independently for purposes of this examination

---

BOX 2.41 TYPES OF GAIT

- Antalgic: where one leg is favoured to the other owing to pain, e.g. in osteoarthritis
- Ataxic: wide based, 'drunken' ± stomping if sensory ataxic, e.g. multiple sclerosis
- Festinating: shuffling, jerky gait, stooped posture, reduced arm swing, difficulty turning and initiating movements, e.g. Parkinson's disease
- Scissoring: lower limbs cross or hit one another, hypertonia and pathological-adduction, e.g. UMN lesions

---

INSPECTION

- Walking aids, e.g. stick, crutches
- Orthotics, e.g. adapted footwear
- Deformity, e.g. hip fixed flexion, leg extension
- Observe for signs of underlying disease, e.g.
  - ○ Tremor, hypomimia (Parkinson's)
  - ○ Nystagmus, staccato speech (cerebellar syndrome)
  - ○ 'Inverse champagne bottle' legs (Charcot–Marie–Tooth)
  - ○ Question mark posture, '*en bloc*' movement (ankylosing spondylitis)

MOVEMENT

- Ask the patient to walk across the room, stop suddenly, turn around and walk back towards you
- Look for:
  - Abnormal arm swing
  - Difficulty stopping and starting
  - Difficulty turning around
  - Abnormal gait (see Box 2.41)

BALANCE

- Ask the patient to perform heel-toe walking – this may intensify any ataxia; note which side the patient tends to fall or lean to
- Ask the patient to balance:
  - On their toes (assesses S1)
  - On their heels (assesses L5)
- Perform Romberg's test asking the patient to:
  - Place their feet together
  - Hold their arms out in front of them
  - If they are able *to do this safely*, ask them to close their eyes

Romberg's positive test: patient is stable with eyes open but unsteady with eyes closed – this is diagnostic of sensory ataxia (caused by peripheral neuropathies or disease processes affecting dorsal columns).

BOX 2.42 CAUSES OF SENSORY ATAXIA

- Demyelinating disease (e.g. multiple sclerosis)
- Sub-acute combined degeneration of the cord
- Tabes dorsalis (syphilis)
- Diabetes mellitus
- Cervical myelopathy
- Friedrich's ataxia

CENTRAL NERVOUS SYSTEM EXAMINATION

INTRODUCTION

- Introduce yourself, explain procedure and request permission
- Enquire about any pain or discomfort
- Ensure adequate lighting (and that it can be turned off)
- Sit opposite patient

INSPECTION
General

- Ptosis

- Strabismus
- Asymmetry
- Facial palsies/weakness
- Swelling
- Scars

Cranial nerve I – olfactory

- Ask patient if they have noticed any change in their sense of smell
- Assess with formally scented bottles if indicated (rarely performed)

Cranial nerve II – optic

(Mnemonic 'AFRO'.)

- A – acuity (with glasses if normally worn): Snellen chart and colour vision (Ishihara charts)
- F – fields: assess by confrontation (see p. 92)
- R – reflexes: assess light and accommodation reflex is intact
- O – ophthalmoscopy including red reflex (see p. 88)

Cranial nerves III, IV, VI

- Nystagmus/diplopia
- Accommodation/pupillary reflexes/convergence

Cranial nerve III – oculomotor nerve

- Motor supply to the extraocular muscles: medial, superior and inferior rectus and inferior oblique
- Assess eye movement by asking patient to follow a pen or hat pin in an 'H' shape, i.e. vertical, horizontal and diagonal
- Ask if there is any diplopia on the extremes of gaze
- Note any nystagmus and its direction. Remember that nystagmus on extreme lateral gaze is a normal variant

Cranial nerve IV – trochlear nerve

- Supplies the superior oblique muscle

Cranial nerve VI – abducens nerve

- Supplies the lateral rectus muscle

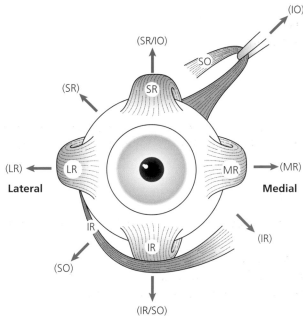

MR: medical rectus
SR: superior rectus
LR: lateral rectus
IR: inferior rectus
SO: superior oblique
IO: inferior oblique

→ Direction of movement of globe by muscle in brackets

Figure 2.7 Extrinsic eye muscles and their movements

Cranial nerve V – trigeminal nerve

- Sensory:
    - This nerve has three branches, all of which provide sensation to the face

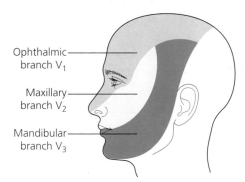

Figure 2.8 Sensory dermatomes of the trigeminal nerve

    - Assess light touch and pin prick in all three areas
    - Assess the corneal reflex laterally with a wisp of cotton wool
- Motor:
    - It also supplies motor fibres to the masseter, temporalis and pterygoid muscle
    - Assess masseter and temporalis tone ('grit teeth')

- Move jaw from side to side (pterygoids)
- Perform the jaw jerk:
    - Ask the patient to slightly open their mouth
    - Place your finger on the chin
    - Gently strike your finger with the tendon hammer – exaggerated opening of the mouth in response to this is pathological

Cranial nerve VII – facial nerve

- Sensory:
    - The facial nerve supplies taste to the anterior two-thirds of the tongue. It can be tested with formal tastes, e.g. salt
- Motor – to the facial muscles:
    - Observe patient for any asymmetry or tics
    - Ask patient to screw eyes up tightly, clench teeth, puff out cheeks, smile, whistle and elevate eyebrows – resist these movements to assess power

Note: Due to bilateral innervation in UMN lesions the function of the upper face is preserved, i.e. both sides of the forehead frontalis muscle will rise. Only one side will rise in a LMN lesion.

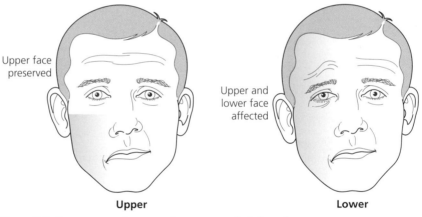

Upper face preserved

Upper and lower face affected

Upper   **Lower**

Figure 2.9 Upper versus lower motor neurone facial weakness

BOX 2.43 CAUSES OF FACIAL NERVE PALSY

UMN:	LMN:
• Multiple sclerosis	• Bell's palsy
• Cerebrovascular events	• Myasthenia gravis
• Space-occupying lesions	• Myotonic dystrophy
	• Sarcoidosis
	• Guillain–Barré syndrome
	• Local trauma
	• Parotid disease

Cranial nerve VIII – vestibulocochlear nerve

This nerve has two main parts as the name suggests.

- Vestibular branch – controls balance and posture:
  - Doll's eyes reflex (with patient lying down)
- Cochlear branch – supplies hearing:
  - Gross assessment of hearing – cover and whisper a number in each ear alternately, asking the patient to repeat it
  - Rinne's test – place a vibrating 256 Hz or 512 Hz tuning fork in air next to ear and against mastoid bone (see p. 94)
  - Weber's test – place vibrating tuning fork in the centre of the forehead (see p. 95)

BOX 2.44 CAUSES OF HEARING LOSS

There are three types of hearing loss to consider.

Conductive:
- Otitis externa, foreign bodies, wax
- Chronic otitis media
- Trauma
- Syndromes, e.g. Marfan's

Sensorineural:
- Genetic – Usher's, Klippel–Feil syndrome
- Measles, mumps, rubella
- Prematurity
- Meningitis
- B vitamin deficiency
- Multiple sclerosis

Mixed

Cranial nerve IX and X – glossopharyngeal nerve and vagus nerve

These two nerves are best examined together as they have overlapping motor and sensory functions. Examine:

- Patient's voice quality
- Say 'ahh' – note equal elevation of soft palate and uvula (this will deviate away from the side of any lesion)
- Offer to assess gag reflex

Cranial nerve XI – accessory nerve

This motor nerve supplies the sternocleidomastoid and trapezius muscles.

- Ask the patient to turn their head to the left and right against your hands
- Ask the patient to shrug their shoulders against your hands

Cranial nerve XII – hypoglossal nerve

This motor nerve supplies the tongue. Ask the patient to:

- Stick out their tongue: note any fasciculation, deviation and abnormality in muscle bulk
- Move it left and right
- Push against inside of mouth against resistance

FURTHER INVESTIGATIONS (see p. 80)

- Blood tests – to assess infection, renal or liver abnormality, thyroid dysfunction
- Lumbar puncture – to assess, e.g. multiple sclerosis (oligoclonal bands), meningitis (white cell count, organisms)
- Imaging – CT head or MRI for space-occupying or vascular lesions
- Electroencephalography (EEG) – to assess any epileptiform activity

OPHTHALMOSCOPY

Examination of the fundi using ophthalmoscopy or fundoscopy can reveal a vast amount of information about underlying disease processes.

INTRODUCTION

- Introduce yourself and explain procedure and request permission
- Enquire about any pain or discomfort
- Ensure adequate lighting (and that it can be turned off)
- Seat patient opposite yourself
- Warn patient you will be coming very close to them and that the light will be very bright

PREPARATION

- Ensure the ophthalmoscope light is white and bright
- Correct the magnification to correspond with your eyesight
- Ask the patient if they wear glasses or contact lenses

EXAMINATION

- Ask the patient to focus on a distant object (even if you get in their way)
- Assess the red reflex from about 1 m away – observe the eyes in turn
- Place your hand on the patient's shoulder or forehead to guide yourself towards their eye, without knocking into them
- While looking through the ophthalmoscope, gradually move closer to the patient's eye at a diagonal of 15°

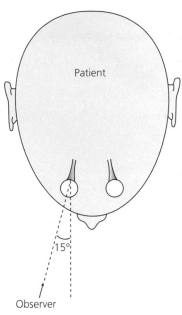

Figure 2.10 Angle of examination to locate disc

- The retina should come into focus at about 2 cm from the eye
- The optic disc should then become visible – a yellow disc with overlying blood vessels
- Observe the disc for:
    - Sharpness of margins
    - Colour of the disc
    - Width of the physiological cup
- Follow the main vessels to the peripheries observing:
    - Calibre
    - Width (arterioles are two-thirds the width of veins)
    - Beading
    - Strictures
- Check the peripheries for: dots and blots, haemorrhages, exudates
- Finally ask the patient to look straight at the light to assess the macula

BOX 2.45 COMMON FUNDOSCOPY FINDINGS

Diabetic retinopathy

Background:
Haemorrhage:
- Leakage of blood into the retina
- Dot, blot, flame-shaped haemorrhages

Oedema:
- Leakage of fluid (transudate)
- Diabetic macular oedema (can occur even in background disease)

Microaneurysms:
- Outpouchings in venous end of capillaries
- Earliest sign of retinopathy, found in the central macula

Exudates:
- Leakage of lipid
- Yellowish deposits, usually in the macula

Pre-proliferative changes:
Cotton wool spots:
- With blockage of fine retinal capillaries a feathery whitish area is produced called a 'cotton wool spot' – this represents a focal infarct

Vein abnormalities:
- Characterize an ischaemic retina
- Venous looping, beading and engorgement can be seen

Proliferative:
- Neovascularization
- Photocoagulation scars
- Cataracts

Hypertensive retinopathy
- Silver wiring (thickened arterioles)
- Arteriovenous nipping
- Cotton wool spots, hard exudates
- Flame haemorrhages
- Disc swelling

Papilloedema
- Tortuous, dilated veins
- Swollen, hyperaemic discs with blurred margins
- Loss of venous pulsation (a difficult sign)

Optic atrophy
- Very pale, featureless discs

PUPIL EXAMINATION

Examination of the pupils is a quick and easy part of the CNS examination. It can potentially yield a large amount of important information.

PUPILLARY REFLEXES

Direct and consensual light reflex

- Seat patient in a darkened room
- Shine a bright light at one eye
- Both pupils should constrict
  - The eye in which the light was shone constricts as part of the direct light reflex
  - The other eye is responding as part of the consensual light reflex

Accommodation reflex

- Seat the patient in a well-lit room
- Ask them to look at a distant point
- Then ask them to look at a near object (~10 cm away)
- Convergence of the eyes should be accompanied by bilateral pupillary constriction

---

BOX 2.46 COMMON PUPILLARY ABNORMALITIES

Miosis (small pupil)
- Argyll Robertson pupil – bilateral constricted pupils, irregular, accommodation intact, no response to light (due to diabetes or syphilis)
- Anisocoria – unilateral variant of the normal population
- Old age – reflexes intact
- Horner's syndrome – interruption of the sympathetic innervation of the eye causing a small pupil on the affected side and a partial ptosis
- Drugs, e.g. opiates

Mydriasis (large pupil)
- Holmes–Adie pupil – idiopathic, accommodation reflex intact, sluggish response to light, associated with absent reflexes
- Third nerve palsy – dilated pupil, eye looking 'down and out', complete ptosis
- Drugs, e.g. cocaine, atropine

SWINGING LIGHT TEST

- Swinging the torch from eye to eye should induce immediate constriction bilaterally
- This signifies that the normal direct and the consensual light reflex are intact
- However, with a relative afferent pupillary defect (RAPD) or Marcus Gunn pupil, the following occurs:
  - Light on the affected eye causes a **slow** direct reflex and consensual reflex (i.e. the afferent fibres in this eye are affected)
  - Light on the normal eye causes a **normal** direct reflex and consensual reflex (i.e. the afferent fibres and reflexes in the good eye are *not* affected)

○　While swinging the light from the normal eye back to the affected eye dilation occurs in both eyes

○　When the light reaches the affected eye again this dilation is faster than the sluggish constriction (described above), i.e. the affected eye dilates as the light is being swung quickly into it

VISUAL FIELDS EXAMINATION

This examination forms part of the CNS examination and tests the integrity of the retina, optic nerve and tracts and occipital cortex.

It is performed by 'confrontation' and all patients should go on for formal field testing (perimetry) if defects are found.

INTRODUCTION

- Introduce yourself and explain procedure and request permission
- Enquire about visual symptoms
- Ensure adequate lighting and black-out blinds
- Ensure patient is seated comfortably

INSPECTION

Fields

- Sit directly opposite patient
- Ask: 'Can you see my whole face?'
- Ask the patient to cover one eye with their hand
- Cover your opposite eye with your hand
- Ask the patient to look at your nose
- Using a wiggling finger or hat pin to examine the outer visual fields
- Bring your hand in diagonally from all four areas of the peripheries (see Fig. 2.11)
- Ask the patient to say immediately when they see your hand
- Note where the patient's fields differ from yours
- Map as shown in Figure 2.12

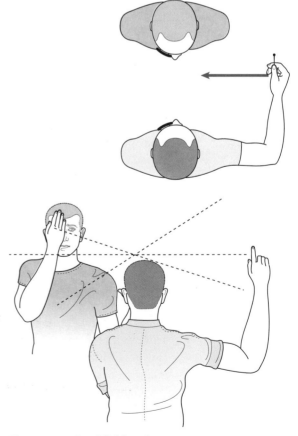

Figure 2.11 Visual field testing

Blind spot and central scotomas

- With one eye remaining closed ask the patient to look at your nose
- Slowly bring in a red hat pin to the centre of the patient's fields
- Ask when it is no longer red or disappears

Inattention

- Ask patient to open both eyes and look at your nose
- Wiggle both your index fingers in the peripheries bilaterally
- Vary between both, one or neither
- Ask patient to point at which side moves or say neither or both

Interpreting field defects

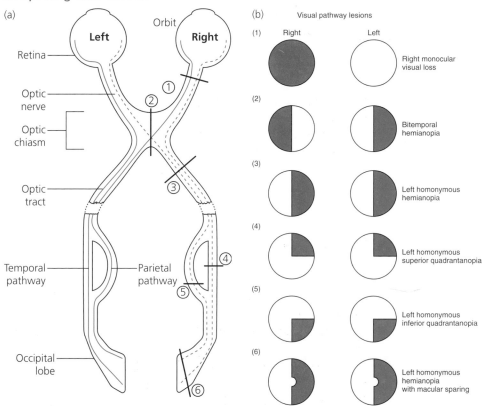

Figure 2.12 (a) Visual pathways and (b) common patterns of visual pathway lesions

- Optic nerve – unilateral field defect
- Optic chiasm – bitemporal hemianopia
- Optic tract – homonymous hemianopia
- Temporal lobe – upper quadrantanopia
- Parietal lobe – lower quadrantanopia
- Occipital lobe – homonymous hemianopia (sparing macula)

BOX 2.47 DIFFERENTIAL DIAGNOSES OF FIELD DEFECTS

- Vascular disease
- Pituitary tumour (bitemporal hemianopia)
- Cerebral neoplasm
- Multiple sclerosis (optic neuritis)
- Haemorrhage
- Abscesses
- Sarcoidosis
- Retinal artery embolus

INVESTIGATIONS

- Formal perimetry
- Cross-sectional imaging

RINNE'S AND WEBER'S TESTS

Rinne's and Weber's tests are key in assessing the type and potential causes of deafness.

BACKGROUND

- Both tests use a tuning fork to assess hearing. To make a tuning fork vibrate, pinch the two prongs together firmly and release

RINNE'S TEST

- A vibrating tuning fork (either 256 Hz or 512 Hz) is placed firstly on the mastoid process until the sound is no longer heard
- Then it is placed next to the ear, where the sound should become audible again
- This is the normal result, a positive test, whereby air conduction (AC) is better than bone conduction (BC)
- In conductive hearing loss, BC is better than AC: a negative Rinne's test result
- In sensorineural hearing loss both BC and AC will be diminished to roughly the same degree, therefore giving a positive result

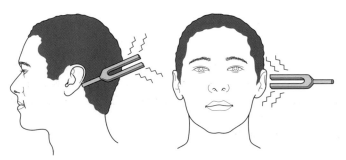

Figure 2.13 Rinne's test

WEBER'S TEST

- This test elicits a sensorineural hearing loss
- A vibrating tuning fork is placed in the centre of a patient's forehead, with their eyes closed
- The patient is asked in which ear the note is heard louder
- Normally, it should be equal bilaterally
- If there is conductive hearing loss the sound is heard loudest in the affected ear. (This may be because this ear does not receive the normal ambient sounds too, owing to the obstruction, or that this obstruction amplifies the sound transmitted by the bone)
- If there is sensorineural hearing loss the sound is best heard in the unaffected ear

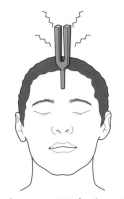

Figure 2.14 Weber's test

Table 2.2

Rinne	Weber (N)	Weber louder Ⓛ	Weber louder Ⓡ
Both AC > BC	N	SN loss Ⓡ	SN loss Ⓛ
Ⓛ BC > AC	–	C loss Ⓛ	–
Ⓡ BC > AC	–	–	C loss Ⓡ

Key: Ⓛ = left; Ⓡ = right; AC = air conduction; BC = bone conduction; SN = Sensorineural; C = Conductive; N = normal.

SPEECH AND LANGUAGE

Assessment of a patient's speech and use of language can provide valuable clues as to the nature and location of neurological lesions.

INTRODUCTION

- Introduce yourself
- Explain procedure
- Request permission

SPEECH

- Normal speech – ask the patient questions with easy answers such as: 'What did you have for breakfast?', 'What is your name and address?' Ensure that the patient understands what you are saying before continuing further. Listen for:
  - Slurring of speech
  - Difficulty word-finding
  - Neologisms
  - Staccato speech (cerebellar syndrome)

- Articulation – ask them to repeat after you:
  - 'British constitution'
  - 'West Register Street'
  - 'Red lorry, yellow lorry' (lingual sounds)
  - 'Baby hippopotamus' (labial sounds)
- Comprehension – assesses types of dysphasia:
  - Expressive – ask them:
    - Their name
    - Their address
    - Their date of birth
  - Receptive – ask them to:
    - Put out your tongue
    - Point to the ceiling
    - Shut your eyes
  - More complicated:
    - Pick up the paper, fold it in half, place it under the table
  - Nominal – ask them to name:
    - Watch: the hands, the winder
    - Pen
    - A comb
  - If unable to name them, give them possibilities/options
    - 'Is this a pen, comb or watch?' – patient may correctly say yes/no
- Phonics (assesses bulbar abnormality) – ask them to repeat after you:
  - Mm mm mm (VII nerve)
  - K k k (IX, X nerves)
  - La la la (XII nerve)
- Language:
  - Ask patient to write a sentence
  - Ask patient to read out loud

BOX 2.48 COMMON SPEECH ABNORMALITIES

Dysarthria – inability to articulate words correctly, e.g. slurring of speech
- May occur secondary to a wide range of lesions e.g. cerebellar disease, strokes (UMN), bulbar palsies (LMN), extrapyramidal lesions

Dysphonia – impaired phonation due laryngeal lesions, e.g. vagal nerve damage

Dysphasia – impairment of expression or comprehension
- Expressive (Broca's area lesion – frontal lobe, dominant hemisphere) Comprehends but cannot express
- Receptive (Wernicke's area lesion – temporal lobe, dominant hemisphere) Unable to comprehend questions
- Global (damage to both areas) – unable to comprehend or express
- Nominal – unable to name objects

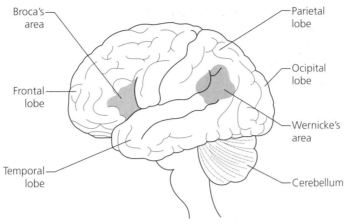

Figure 2.15 Broca's and Wernicke's areas

FOLLOW UP

- Full neurological history and examination
- Mini-mental State Examination
- Blood tests (see p. 80)
- Imaging (see p. 80)

MENTAL STATE

There are several methods of assessing a patient's mental state: these are useful tools in assessing cognitive function.

Note: patients for whom English is not their first language may not reach a score indicative of their actual cognitive state.

ABBREVIATED MENTAL TEST SCORE (AMTS)

As the name suggests this abbreviated test is a rapid tool for assessing cognitive state. This test should be memorized.

The maximum score is 10 and a score <7 suggests significant cognitive impairment.

- What is your age? (1 point)
- What is your date of birth? (1 point)
- What year are we in? (1 point)
- What time of day is it? (1 point)
- Where are we? (1 point)
- Who is the current monarch? (1 point)
- When was the second world war? (1 point)
- Count backwards from 20 to 1 (1 point)
- Recognize two people, e.g. a doctor and a nurse (1 point)
- Recall a three-part address: 50 West Street (1 point)

MINI-MENTAL STATE EXAMINATION (MMSE)

This more detailed test is scored out of 30 and is performed with the help of a pro forma:

- 25–30: normal
- 18–24: mild–moderate impairment
- <17: indicates severe impairment

Orientation

- What is the:
  - Day
  - Date
  - Month
  - Year
  - Season?

(1 for each, maximum 5 points)

- Which:
  - Floor
  - Hospital
  - Street
  - Town
  - Country are we in?

(1 for each, maximum 5 points)

Registration

- Slowly name three everyday objects, e.g. apple, table, penny
- Ask the patient to repeat the three objects back to you (1 point each)
- Repeat the objects up to six times until they are learned – record how many times this takes

Attention and calculation

Either:

- Ask the patient to spell WORLD backwards (1 point for each letter in the correct position – maximum 5 points)

Or:

- Ask the patient to count backwards from 100 in sevens, e.g. 100, 93, 86, 79, 72 and 65 ('serial 7s') (1 point for each correct answer – with respect to the previous number, 5 maximum)

Recall

- Ask the patient to recall the three items you named earlier: apple, table and penny (1 point each, maximum 3 points)

Language

- Ask the patient to name two objects you point to, e.g. a pencil and a watch (1 point each, maximum 2 points)
- Ask the patient to repeat *once*: 'No ifs, ands or buts' (1 attempt and 1 point only)
- Three-stage command: ask the patient to:
  - Pick up a piece of paper with their left hand
  - Fold it in half
  - Place it on the floor

(1 point each, 3 point maximum)

- Write 'Close your eyes' clearly on a piece of paper and ask the patient to read out the instructions and follow the command (1 point only)
- Ask the patient to write a short sentence. It must include a subject and a verb and make sense, although spelling and punctuation are unimportant (1 point only)
- Show the patient a picture of two pentagons that intersect, forming a quadrangle (see Figure 2.16) and ask them to copy them (to gain 1 mark two intersecting pentagons must be drawn)

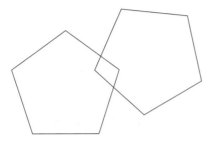

Figure 2.16 Two intersecting pentagons

OTOSCOPY

Examination of the ear is an important skill, especially in primary care where patients presenting with ear, nose and throat symptoms are common.

All children with systemic upset or fever should have their ears examined as otitis media is a common cause.

INTRODUCTION
- Introduce yourself, explain procedure and request permission
- Enquire about any pain or discomfort
- Ensure the light on the otoscope is working
- Select an appropriate speculum for the ear size
- Seat the patient and stand to the side of them

THE OUTER EAR
First examine the outer ear for any obvious signs of disease:

- Cauliflower ears
- Gouty tophi
- Vesicles around the ear, the face or in the canal (Ramsey Hunt syndrome)

OTOSCOPY
- The otoscope should be held in the hand that corresponds to the ear being examined
- It should be held between the thumb and forefingers, with the base pointing towards the ceiling, like a pen
- The other hand should simultaneously gently pull the ear upwards and backwards

EAR CANAL

Note any:

- Eczema – dry, flaky skin
- Erythema, trauma (e.g. from cotton buds)
- Rash (e.g. vesicles)
- Wax
- Foreign body (common in children)
- Inflamed, swollen canal ± discharge – otitis externa

EAR DRUM

Normally this appears a pearly-grey colour with the vertical malleus and a cone of reflected light being visible. Common abnormalities include:

- A hole (perforation) in the eardrum
- Grommets (surgically inserted drainage tubes)
- Acute infection of the middle ear (acute otitis media) – yellow, red, pus, bulging membrane
- Cholesteatoma (pearly white mass)

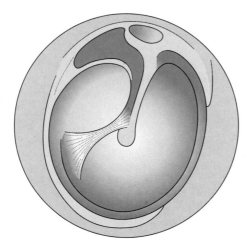

Figure 2.17 Normal eardrum at otoscopy

PARKINSON'S DISEASE

This devastating disease comprises a combination of poverty of movement, rigidity, tremor and postural instability. It is caused by degeneration of the dopaminergic neurones in the substantia nigra. Its aetiology is poorly understood and may be mimicked by several other disease processes that cause parkinsonism.

KEY CHARACTERISTICS

- Daily fluctuation in severity
- Symptoms start in the upper limbs
- Asymmetrical presentation (e.g. unilateral loss of arm swing)

INTRODUCTION

- Explain the examination
- Ask about painful areas
- Request permission
- Position patient
- Expose arms and legs

INSPECTION

Gait

- Festinating gait – shuffling steps
- Forward flexed posture
- Difficulty initiating movements ('freezing') and turning
- Lack of arm swing
- Abnormal righting reflex

Arms

- Resting tremor:
  - Unilateral or asymmetric distribution
  - Most conspicuous at rest
  - 'pill-rolling'
  - 3–5 Hertz
  - Exacerbated by distraction, e.g. tapping other hand on knee
  - Improved by concentration
- 'Cogwheeling' tone at wrist and – tremor superimposed on increased tone and 'lead-pipe' rigidity at the elbow
- Difficulty with rhythmical movements and bradykinesia – slowly and inefficiently opposing each finger to the thumb
- Micrographia – request sample of handwriting

Face and head

- Facial hypomimia – expressionless face
- Titubation
- Slow blink rate
- Absent glabellar tap
- Speech is quiet and monotonous
- Dysphagia
- Drooling
- Intellectual deterioration occurs late in one-third

BOX 2.49 PARKINSON'S TRIAD OF SYMPTOMS

Asymmetrical onset of:
- Bradykinesia
- Rigidity
- Tremor

INVESTIGATIONS

- Postural blood pressure (autonomic neuropathy of multisystem atrophy)
- CT brain

BOX 2.50 CAUSES OF PARKINSONISM

- Parkinson's disease
- Vascular dementia
- Supranuclear palsy
- Multisystem atrophy
- Lewy body dementia
- Wilson's disease
- Hypoparathyroidism
- Normal pressure hydrocephalus

MANAGEMENT

- Social:
  - Home adaptation with occupational therapy input
- Medical:
  - L-dopa
  - Dopamine agonists: bromocriptine, pergolide, apomorphine
- Surgical:
  - Basal ganglia ablation
  - Deep brain stimulation

STROKE

Stroke is the third most common cause of death in the UK and a quoted 11 000 people have a stroke per year in the UK (www.nhs.uk).

There are two broad categories:

- Ischaemic: caused by interruption or occlusion of the vascular supply to the brain
- Haemorrhagic: caused by ischaemia and the pressure effect of intracranial bleeding, following injury to the vascular supply

---

BOX 2.51 RISK FACTORS FOR STROKE

Ischaemic:
- Cerebrovascular disease: smoking, diabetes, hypertension, obesity
- Atrial fibrillation
- Patent foramen ovale
- Carotid artery stenosis
- Cardiac valvular dysfunction or prostheses
- Oral contraceptive pill
- Vasculitis
- Nephrotic syndrome

Haemorrhagic:
- Hypertension
- Anticoagulation
- Alcoholic liver disease
- Head injury/trauma
- Space-occupying lesion, i.e. haematoma, abscess, neoplasm
- Berry aneurysm (polycystic kidneys)
- Arteriovenous malformations

HISTORY

- UMN weakness:
  - Predominantly unilateral
  - Upper and/or lower limb
- Sensory impairment – predominantly unilateral
- Speech impairment
  - Dysarthria
  - Dysphasia: receptive/expressive (see p. 96)
- Facial asymmetry:
  - Drooling
  - Asymmetrical smile
- Dysphagia
- Impaired vision/visual field defect
- Ataxia, collapse/falls
- Severe headache, e.g. 'thunder-clap' headache in subarachnoid haemorrhage
- Loss of continence
- Cognitive impairment
- Loss of consciousness (rare)

BOX 2.52 RECOGNIZING STROKE AND SUMMONING HELP: 'FAST' METHOD

- F – facial weakness, asymmetry
- A – arm weakness, numbness
- S – slurring or difficulty understanding a patient's speech
- T – time: quick recognition and thrombolytic treatment may save lives

---

Examination

- The key to diagnosing a stroke is in the recognition of a UMN lesion, along with the other cardinal features
- The severity of symptoms depend on the exact location of the vascular deficit and the cerebral area it supplies

Face

- Weakness of the muscles of the face causing asymmetry – contralateral to the lesion
  - Note: the periorbital and forehead muscles will be spared (if they are also involved this represents an LMN deficit)
- Hemisensory loss – contralateral to the lesion (see Figure 2.9, p. 86)
- Drooling

Eyes

- Homonymous hemianopia (bilateral field defect on confrontation)

Speech (see p. 95)

- Dysarthria: slurring of speech
- Dysphasia
- Receptive: unable to comprehend

- Expressive: able to understand but not express

Swallow
- Dysphagia and a resultant poor swallow results from bulbar muscle involvement
- This puts the patient at high risk of aspiration

Limbs
- Inspection: normal (often the case initially) or arm held in flexion, leg held in extension
- Tone: normal (initially) or increased
- Power: reduced (unilateral weakness)
- Reflexes: hyperreflexia, extensor plantar (predominantly unilateral)
- Sensation: hemisensory disturbance or loss (predominantly unilateral)
- Coordination: reduced in affected limbs
- Other signs include:
  - Cerebellar signs, e.g. nystagmus – suggestive of brainstem/cerebellar involvement
  - Agnosias: visual, auditory, tactile

INVESTIGATIONS
- Baseline blood tests including clotting studies, autoimmune screen and blood glucose (see p. 80)
- Blood pressure
- ECG
- Echocardiogram
- Carotid Doppler to look for carotid stenosis (potential source of embolus)
- CT brain: may be normal in ischaemic acute setting, but will show location of lesions/deficit when performed some hours later. Most useful for ruling out haemorrhage
- MRI brain: more detailed, sensitive imaging

TREATMENT
- Ischaemic stroke:
  - Aspirin
  - Dipyridamole in addition if recurrent events on aspirin alone
  - Thrombolysis (if meets criteria and recognized early)
  - Blood pressure control
  - Statins
  - Carotid endarterectomy (if > 70% stenosis)
- Haemorrhagic stroke:
  - Reversal of anticoagulation
  - Radiologically guided aneurysm coiling
  - Neurosurgical intervention, i.e. surgery
- Admission to a stroke unit:
  - Evidence suggests that outcome is improved in a specialist environment
- Rehabilitation:
  - This is an integral part of stroke recovery and not only involves medical input but also incorporates physiotherapy, speech therapy, dieticians and occupational and psychotherapists

TRANSIENT ISCHAEMIC ATTACKS

- Transient ischaemic attacks (TIAs) exhibit the symptoms of a stroke, but resolve quickly, typically in less than 24 hours. The definition of TIA is changing as early, more aggressive treatments of ischaemic neurological events are being used
- They may herald a full stroke, within the subsequent month, in up to 20 per cent of patients
- Full investigation and treatment of risk factors is essential to prevent this

MULTIPLE SCLEROSIS

Multiple sclerosis is a debilitating disease affecting the central nervous system. It commonly presents in young to middle-aged adults, more often females.

BOX 2.53 TYPES OF MULTIPLE SCLEROSIS

- Relapsing-remitting: alternating attacks and recovery periods
- Primary-progressive: continuously worsening, no discrete attacks or recovery
- Secondary-progressive: progressive after an initial relapsing/remitting course
- Progressive-relapsing: progressive course with attacks of worsening function

---

HISTORY

- Ophthalmic pain, impaired/loss of vision (optic neuritis)
- Myalgia
- Limb weakness, spasm, pain, numbness
- Urinary/bladder dysfunction
- Erectile dysfunction
- Lethargy, malaise
- Depression

INSPECTION

- General:
  - Typically young female patient
  - A wheelchair or walking aid may be present
  - Patient may be catheterized (often long term)
- Peripheral nervous system examination:
  - Typically produces a spastic paraparesis
  - Inspect: look for signs of UMN disease, e.g. upper limb flexion, lower limb extension
  - Tone: increased (spasticity), clonus
  - Power: reduced
  - Reflexes: brisk, upgoing plantars
  - Sensory deficit
  - Coordination: diminished

- ○ Dorsal column signs may also be evident, e.g.:
    - ♦ Gait disturbance
    - ♦ Positive Romberg's test
    - ♦ Impaired proprioception and vibration sense
- Cerebellar examination – cerebellar signs are common in multiple sclerosis. These include:
    - ♦ Dysdiadochokinesis
    - ♦ Dysmetria (finger overshoot)
    - ♦ Ataxia
    - ♦ Nystagmus
    - ♦ Intention tremor
    - ♦ Slurred or staccato speech

EYE EXAMINATION

- Optic nerve damage (five signs):
    - ○ Decreased visual acuity
    - ○ Impaired colour vision
    - ○ Optic atrophy (pale discs)
    - ○ Central scotoma
    - ○ Relative afferent papillary defect
- Internuclear ophthalmoplegia
    - ○ Seen while examining saccades
    - ○ The adducting (abnormal) eye is slow on lateral gaze with the abducted one moving quickly and seeming to 'encourage' the slow one with jerky nystagmus
    - ○ May be bilateral
- Nystagmus
- Ptosis

INVESTIGATIONS

- Cerebrospinal fluid examination – oligoclonal bands (present in over 80 per cent of patients)
- MRI scan – periventricular white matter lesions
- Visual evoked potentials – prolonged signal time

TREATMENT

- Multidisciplinary team approach including physiotherapy, occupational therapy, psychological support, acupuncture, aromatherapy
- Analgesia
- Systemic steroids – reduces duration of attacks, does not affect disease progression
- Disease-modifying agents, i.e. interferon beta – reduces number of relapses

MYASTHENIA GRAVIS

This autoimmune disease affects 1 in 10 000 people in the UK, predominantly young women and elderly men. Autoantibodies are formed against postsynaptic nicotinic acetylcholine receptors of the neuromuscular junction. More than three-quarters of cases are associated with thymic abnormalities and other autoimmune diseases.

HISTORY

Patients are likely to present with symptoms of muscle fatigue which worsens on repetition and improves on rest.

Symptoms and signs include:

- Diplopia and ptosis
- Strabismus
- Facial muscle weakness (expressionless, snarling smile)
- Dysphagia, dysarthria
- Proximal muscle weakness
- Reduced exercise tolerance
- Inability to maintain posture or neck extension
- Respiratory weakness and failure

EXAMINATION

- Speech and swallowing: bulbar muscle weakness
- Ptosis – worsens on looking up
- Complex ophthalmoplegia
- Cannot whistle
- Voice weak (diminishes on counting out loud) and nasal
- Upper and lower limb weakness
- Reflexes exaggerated (or normal)

INVESTIGATIONS

- Antinicotinic acetylcholine receptor antibodies (ARA) in 90 per cent
- Tensilon test: weakness improves with edrophonium injection (anti-cholinesterase inhibitor). Note: need crash trolley nearby – may induce arrhythmias and asystole
- Respiratory function monitoring, i.e. blood gas analysis, PEFR, FVC
- Chest X-ray: for aspiration pneumonia as aspiration risk
- CT thorax or MRI to rule out thymoma
- Electromyography (EMG) – to confirm the diagnosis

TREATMENT

- Anticholinesterase inhibitors (e.g. pyridostigmine)
- Thymectomy (for thymoma) – 10 per cent will improve
- Steroids
- Azathioprine

BOX 2.54 ASSOCIATED AUTOIMMUNE DISEASES

Hypothyroidism	Rheumatoid arthritis	Pernicious anaemia
Thyrotoxicosis	Systemic lupus erythematosus	Sjögren's syndrome
Diabetes mellitus	Sarcoidosis	Polymyalgia rheumatica

CEREBELLAR SYNDROME

This syndrome comprises a unique collection of features even though it is caused by a wide range of disease processes.

INTRODUCTION

- Explain the examination
- Ask about painful areas
- Request permission
- Position patient
- Expose arms and legs

EXAMINATION

If cerebellar symptoms are noted on neurological examination then the mnemonic 'DANISH' will aid eliciting further features:

- **D** – Dysdiadochokinesis:
  - This is difficulty in performed rapid, alternating movements, e.g. tapping the palm on one hand with the palmar and dorsal of the fingers of the other
- **A** – Ataxia and wide-based gait:
  - From the Greek meaning 'absence of order', the spinocerebellar form of ataxia manifests as:
    - A wide-based gait, similar to that of alcohol intoxication
    - Heel–shin incoordination
    - Intention tremor
    - Ataxic speech – see below
  - The patient may lurch towards the side of a lesion
  - The foot is often turned outwards
- **N** – Nystagmus:
  - This describes abnormal rhythmical movements of the eye in any direction
  - Often the fast phase of nystagmus is towards the side of a cerebellar lesion
- **I** – Intention tremor with past pointing:
  - This is exhibited with the finger–nose test
  - It occurs on the ipsilateral side of the lesion
  - The tremor represents ataxia of the upper limbs
- **S** – Staccato or slurred speech
  - Ataxic dysarthria occurs with staccato, explosive speech owing to random, uncoordinated movement of the relevant muscles
- **H** – Hypotonia:
  - This may be severe and progressive

INVESTIGATIONS

These are analogous to those for the peripheral and central nervous systems (see p. 80).

MUSCULOSKELETAL

GAIT, ARMS, LEGS, SPINE (GALS) EXAMINATION

This screening tool is valuable in diagnosing gross musculoskeletal disease.

INTRODUCTION
- Explain the examination and request permission
- Ask about painful areas
- Position patient appropriately
- Expose to underwear

THREE INITIAL QUESTIONS
- Do you have any difficulty with dressing or washing yourself?
- Do you have any stiffness or pains in your arms or legs, neck or back?
- Do you have any difficulty with stairs or steps?

INSPECTION

Gait

Ask patient to perform a brief walk.

- Look for:
  - Asymmetry
  - Limping (antalgic)
  - Foot drop
  - Broad based
  - Arm swing
  - Pelvic tilt

Arms
- Look for:
  - Skin changes, scars
  - Swelling
  - Wasting
  - Deformity
  - Nodules (check elbows)
- Feel:
  - Tenderness at metacarpophalangeal (MCP) joints
- Move:
  - Abduction of arms to 180° and touch small of the back
  - Elbow extension
  - Wrist extension and flexion
  - Forearm pronation and supination
  - Pincer grip and agility of fingers

Legs
- Inspect for:
  - Skin changes, scars
  - Swelling
  - Wasting
  - Deformity
- Feel:
  - Squeeze across the MTPs for tenderness
- Move:
  - Bend knee with hand on patella; feel for crepitus (active then passive)
  - Internally rotate hips (ensure knee is bent)
  - Flex, extend, invert and evert the ankle

Spine
- Inspect for:
  - Asymmetry
  - Normal cervical and lumbar lordosis
  - Kyphosis
  - Scoliosis
  - Scars, skin changes
  - Deformity
- Feel:
  - For bony tenderness
- Move:
  - Ask patient to bend forwards and touch their toes; assessing vertebral separation (<15 cm finger to floor distance)
  - Assess lateral flexion of the neck (ear touches shoulder)

HIP EXAMINATION

INTRODUCTION
- Explain examination and gain consent
- Ask patient to remove clothes below waist to underwear
- Offer a chaperone
- Ensure good lighting

INSPECTION
- Observe the patient while standing and lying supine
- Check that the iliac crests are at the same level (see below)
- Examine anteriorly and posteriorly for:
  - Pelvic tilt
  - Symmetry
  - Scoliosis
  - Deformity
  - Swelling

- ○   Scars
- ○   Wasting
- ○   Difference in leg length

PALPATION

- ASIS bilaterally for pelvic tilt
- Greater trochanter for:
  - ○   Swelling
  - ○   Tenderness
  - ○   Temperature

MEASUREMENT

Assess leg lengths:

- True – ASIS to medial malleolus (with legs parallel)
  - ○   If unequal flex knee to 90° with feet together
  - ○   A higher knee indicates a longer tibia
  - ○   The knee projecting further forward indicates a longer femur
- Apparent – xiphisternum to medial malleolus
  - ○   Not due to bony inequality but abduction/adduction deformity at the hip joint or pelvic tilt

MOVEMENT

- Assess both active and passive range of movements
- Flexion: stabilize pelvis with forearm across both anterior iliac spines and flex hip with knee flexed (~130°)
- Abduction: stabilize pelvis with pressure on contralateral ASIS (~45°)
- Adduction: cross one leg over the other while stabilizing pelvis with a hand on ipsilateral ASIS (~25°)
- Rotation: flex hip and knee to 90° and move tibia to measure internal (~45°) and external rotation (~60°)
- Extension: lie patient prone and extend hip (~15°)
- Assess the patient's gait

MANOEUVRES

- Thomas's test – assesses presence of fixed flexion deformity of hip
  - ○   Place a hand under lumbar spine and flex both hips until small of back is flat on your hand
  - ○   Ask patient to hold one knee and straighten the other leg
  - ○   This leg staying slightly raised off the bed corresponds to the degree of fixed flexion deformity
  - ○   Repeat for other leg
- Trendelenburg test – this detects weakness in hip abductors (mostly commonly due to osteoarthritis)
  - ○   Stand facing patient
  - ○   Hold patient's hands to ensure balance

○ Ask patient to stand on one leg then the other
○ Pelvis on non-weightbearing side should normally tilt upwards with action of ipsilateral abductors
○ With weakness the pelvis tilts down on the non-weightbearing side (positive test)

INVESTIGATIONS

- FBC, inflammatory markers (including ESR)
- Autoantibody screen, e.g. for rheumatoid arthritis
- Arthrocentesis if effusion present
- Plain X-ray
- Ultrasound scan
- MRI

FOLLOW-UP

- Examine knees and lumbar spine (i.e. the joint above and below) – pathology at these sites may be the cause of hip pain
- Examine other joints for signs of systemic arthropathy

BOX 2.55 CAUSES OF HIP PAIN

Children:
- Septic arthritis: more common in children under 5 years
- Transient synovitis (irritable hip): 3–10 year olds
- Perthes' disease: avascular necrosis of femoral head in 4–10 year olds
- Slipped upper femoral epiphysis (SUFE): often obese 10–16 year olds

Adults:
- Osteoarthritis: hip, knee, lumbar spine, sacroiliac joints
- Rheumatoid arthritis (and other seropositive arthropathies)
- Seronegative arthropathy, e.g. ankylosing spondylitis (see p. 133)
- Septic arthritis
- Osteomyelitis
- Trauma, e.g. fracture
- Bursitis
- Tendonitis
- Paget's disease
- Neoplasia (usually metastatic)

KNEE EXAMINATION

INTRODUCTION

- Explain examination and gain consent
- Ask patient to remove clothes below waist to underwear
- Offer a chaperone
- Ensure good lighting

INSPECTION

- Gait – ask the patient to walk away and then towards you
- Inspect anteriorly and posteriorly for:
  - Deformity e.g.:
    - Genu varus: bow-legged
    - Genu valgus: knock-kneed
  - Swelling:
    - Effusion
    - Bursitis
    - Baker's cyst (posteriorly)
  - Scars, e.g. total knee replacement
  - Rashes
  - Wasting
  - Asymmetry

PALPATION

Ask the patient to lie supine and start with the unaffected side.

Assess:

- Temperature (compare sides with back of your hand)
- Joint line tenderness (flex knee and systematically palpate all the joint lines)
- Assess any swellings or effusions with the following:
  - Patellar tap test:
    - Fully extend knee
    - Empty the suprapatellar pouch by sliding your hand down the anterior surface of the thigh, towards the knee
    - Maintain this position above the patella
    - Gently push down on patella with two fingers
    - If it depresses and appears to 'bounce' or tap back, this indicates an underlying effusion
  - Bulge test:
    - Fully extend knee
    - Again empty the suprapatellar pouch and continue to apply pressure above the patella
    - Stroke along the medial aspect of knee to also empty the medial compartment
    - Then do the same along the lateral aspect of the knee
    - If an effusion is present a bulge will be noted medially

MOVEMENT

Assess active and passive movement:

- Ask patient to flex knee (active)
- When full active flexion is reached grasp ankle with right hand and test for further passive flexion with gentle pressure towards patient's buttock
- Normal range = 135–145°

- Ask patient to extend the knee
- On passive extension and flexion hold a hand over the knee joint to assess for crepitation

Ligament tests

- Collateral ligaments:
  - Knee fully extended
  - Hold lower leg by clenching ankle between your right arm and chest and stabilizing tibia with right hand
  - Medial collateral ligament:
    - Gently apply pressure from lateral to medial with left hand
  - Lateral collateral ligament:
    - Gently apply pressure from medial to lateral with left hand

The knee joint should not give way or move during these manoeuvres.

- Cruciate ligaments (Draw test):
  - Flex hip to 45° and knee to 90° with feet flat on table (sit on their foot to stabilize leg)
  - Cup both hands around the back of the knee and stabilize tibia by clenching it between your forefingers
  - Push towards patient to test for posterior cruciate instability
  - Pull away from patient to test for anterior cruciate instability
  - If ligaments intact there should be no movement
  - Lachman's test is specifically for anterior cruciate ligament injuries and is essentially the same but with only 20° of flexion and some external rotation of the knee
- McMurray's test: for meniscal injury
  - Flex knee to 45° and hold heel in right hand
  - With left hand flat over patella and knee joint gently extend and flex the knee whilst internally and externally rotating foot
  - Feel for clunk as meniscus catches medially (= medial meniscus) or laterally (= lateral meniscus)
- Patellar apprehension test:
  - Apply pressure on medial aspect of patellar with leg extended and slowly flex knee
  - Lateral movement of patellar causes pain or tensing of quadriceps to prevent movement and pain (apprehension)
  - Indicates patellar subluxation or patello-femoral instability

INVESTIGATIONS

- FBC, inflammatory markers (including ESR)
- Autoantibody screen, e.g. for rheumatoid arthritis
- Arthrocentesis
- Plain X-ray
- Ultrasound scan
- MRI

FOLLOW-UP

- Examine ankles and hips (i.e. the joints above and below) – pathology at these sites may be the cause of knee pain
- Examine other joints for signs of systemic arthropathy

BOX 2.56 CAUSES OF KNEE PAIN

- Osteoarthritis: hip, knee, ankle
- Rheumatoid arthritis (and other seropositive arthropathies)
- Seronegative arthropathy, e.g. ankylosing spondylitis (see p. 133)
- Osteomyelitis
- Septic arthritis
- Trauma, e.g. fracture, patellar dislocation, haemarthrosis
- Bursitis
- Baker's cyst
- Tendonitis

SHOULDER EXAMINATION

INTRODUCTION

- Introduce yourself to the patient
- Explain examination and gain consent
- Ask about pain
- Ask patient to remove clothes from waist up
- Offer a chaperone
- Ensure good lighting

INSPECTION

Front and back for:

- Deformity
  - Winging of scapula: long thoracic nerve damage, serratus anterior paralysis
  - Clavicular deformity: previous fracture
  - Prominent sternoclavicular or acromioclavicular joints: subluxation
- Swelling
  - Effusion
  - Infection
- Skin changes
  - Erythema
  - Rashes
- Scars
- Wasting, e.g. deltoid muscle with axillary nerve damage
- Symmetry

PALPATION

- Temperature
- Assess any swellings
- Assess sensation (e.g. axillary nerve damage causes numbness of the 'regimental badge' area on the lateral shoulder)
- Palpate joint line:
  - Clavicle
  - Anterior glenohumeral joint
  - Acromioclavicular joint
  - Head of humerus in axilla

MOVEMENT

- Stand in front of patient and ask them to mirror your movements (*active*)
- Then gently assist the movements to assess the *passive* limits of movement

Note: The limits of active and passive movement may differ (as seen in painful arc syndrome – see Box 2.57)

  - Abduction (0–170°)
    - Abduct arms bringing hands behind head
  - Adduction (0–50°)
    - Swing hand flexed at elbow across the chest
  - Flexion (0–165°)
    - Flex arms horizontally
  - Extension (0–60°)
    - Bring straight arm directly backwards
  - Internal rotation (0–70°)
    - Bring back of hands to lumbar spine
  - External rotation (0–100°)
    - Flex elbow to 90° and externally rotate arm holding elbow against side

Note: Full painless range of movement is unlikely to be associated with any pathology.

INVESTIGATIONS

- FBC, inflammatory markers (including ESR)
- Autoantibody screen, e.g. for rheumatoid arthritis
- Arthrocentesis
- Plain X-ray
- Ultrasound scan
- MRI

FOLLOW-UP

- Examine neck, elbow and wrist (i.e. the joints above and below) – pathology at these sites may be the cause of shoulder pain
- Examine other joints for signs of systemic arthropathy

BOX 2.57 COMMON CAUSES OF SHOULDER PAIN

Painful arc syndrome
Active movement impaired, passive movement preserved.
Impingement on acromion during abduction caused by:
- Supraspinatus tendonitis
- Acromioclavicular joint osteoarthritis (painful arc >160°)
- Rotator cuff tear (painful arc 60–120°) caused by: supraspinatus – most common (restriction of abduction); infraspinatus or teres minor (lateral rotation restricted); subscapularis (internal rotation restricted)

Treatment:
- Steroid injection
- Coracoacromial decompression
- Tendon repairs

Adhesive capsulitis (frozen shoulder)
Poorly understood aetiology affecting glenohumeral joint
Elderly patients with no history of trauma
Active and passive movements reduced

Treatment:
- Non-steroidal anti-inflammatory drugs (NSAIDs)
- Steroid injection
- Physiotherapy

ELBOW EXAMINATION

INTRODUCTION
- Introduce yourself to the patient
- Explain examination and gain consent
- Ask about pain
- Ask patient to remove clothing to expose upper limbs
- Ensure good lighting

INSPECTION
- Symmetry
- Deformity:
  - Cubitus valgus: increased carrying angle (normally 5–20°)
  - Cubitus varus: decreased carrying angle (this may indicate joint malunion or instability)
- Swelling: effusion visible as swelling in lateral aspect of elbow
- Nodules: rheumatoid nodules common on medial aspect
- Muscle wasting
- Scars: previous surgery

- Skin changes
  - Atrophy from repeated steroid injections
  - Erythema: bursitis/septic arthritis
  - Rash, e.g. psoriasis

PALPATION

- With elbow fully extended palpate:
  - Medial epicondyle: medial border
    - Tender in tennis elbow
  - Olecranon: centrally, posteriorly
    - Very prominent if subluxed
  - Lateral epicondyle: lateral border
    - Tender in golfer's elbow or ulnar collateral ligament tear
  - Radial head: 2 cm distal to lateral epicondyle
  - Radiohumeral joint: between radial head and humerus
    - Tender in osteoarthritis
- With slight flexion palpate:
  - Olecranon fossa (tender with bursitis)
  - Ulnar groove medially (for thickening or tenderness)
- Temperature
- Assess any swellings

MOVEMENT

- Extension (normally 0°)
  - Align arm and forearm in a straight line
  - Decreased in osteoarthritis and rheumatoid arthritis and fractures
  - Hyperextension of the elbow >10° from the horizontal represents hypermobility
    - Examine for hypermobility in other joints (e.g. Ehlers–Danlos syndrome)
- Flexion (145°)
  - Restricted osteoarthritis or malunion of fractures
  - Most activities of daily living only require a range of 60–120°
- Pronation (75°)
- Supination (85°)
  - Assesses proximal and distal radioulnar joints
  - Reduced after fractures of elbow/forearm/wrist, elbow dislocation, osteo- and rheumatoid arthritis

Table 2.3 Assessment of myotomes

Nerve root	Muscle	Test
C5	Deltoid	Abduct arm to horizontal
C6	Biceps	Flex forearm
C7	Triceps	Extend forearm
C8	Flexor carpi minimi	Flex wrist
T1	Dorsal interossei	Spread fingers

BOX 2.58 NERVE DAMAGE OF THE UPPER LIMB

Ulnar nerve damage:
- Causes: medial epicondyle fracture, osteoarthritis, cubitus valgus
- Deformity: 'claw' hand, hypothenar muscle wasting
- Weakness: medial two lumbricals, interossei, medial half of flexor digitorum profundus
- Sensory loss: medial area of palmar surface of hand and medial one and half digits

Radial nerve damage:
- Cause: mid-humeral fractures
- Deformity: wrist drop
- Weakness: wrist extensor weakness
- Sensory loss: dorsal aspect of root of thumb (anatomical snuff box)

Median nerve damage:
- Cause: supracondylar fractures, wrist lacerations
- Deformity: thenar wasting
- Weakness: injury *above* the elbow: reduced wrist flexion and forearm pronation, injury in the hand affects lumbricals, opponens pollicis, abductor pollicis brevis, flexor pollicis brevis
- Sensory loss: lateral two and a half digits

HAND EXAMINATION

INTRODUCTION

- Introduce yourself to patient
- Explain examination and gain consent
- Ask about pain
- Expose to above the elbows
- Place forearms/hands on a pillow
- Ensure lighting is adequate

INSPECTION

Face

- Shiny, tight skin, expressionless, telangiectasia – all systemic sclerosis
- Cushingoid from steroid use (rheumatoid arthritis)
- Acromegalic or hypothyroid facies – carpal tunnel syndrome

Hands

- Rheumatoid arthritis
  - Spongy swelling, pain and stiffness of MCP joints, proximal interphalangeal (PIP) joints and wrists, symmetrically, bilaterally. (Distal interphalangeal [DIP] joints spared)
  - Subluxed/dislocated MCPs lead to ulnar deviation of the fingers

- ○ Boutonnières and swan-neck deformities of fingers
- ○ Z thumbs
- ○ Muscle wasting – especially hypothenar and thenar eminences and interossei
- ○ Others: nodules/tendon thickening, palmar erythema
- Osteoarthritis
  - ○ May or may not be symmetrical
  - ○ Bony/hard swelling of DIP joints (Heberden's nodes) and PIP joints (Bouchard's nodes)
- Systemic sclerosis
  - ○ Tapering, gangrenous fingers
  - ○ Shiny, tight skin
  - ○ Painful calcified nodules (calcinosis)
  - ○ Nail fold vasculitic changes

Nails

- Pitting, clubbing, onycholysis (nail detachment) – seen in psoriatic arthritis
- Nail fold infarcts, splinter haemorrhages (vasculitis)

Skin

- Colour, consistency, rash (e.g. psoriasis)
- Nodules, crease hyperpigmentation

Elbows

- Look for rheumatoid nodules, psoriatic plaques
- Also look for any evidence of potential ulnar nerve injury

PALPATION

- Nodules (on palms and tendons in rheumatoid arthritis), Dupuytren's contracture, calcinosis (systemic sclerosis)
- Joint swelling – soft or bony
- Joint dislocation/laxity

SENSATION

Check relevant sensory dermatomes:

- Ulnar (C8–T1) – medial area of hand, little and half of ring finger
- Median (C6–T1) – palmar area of lateral hand, index, middle and other half of ring finger
- Radial (C6–8) – over first dorsal interossei

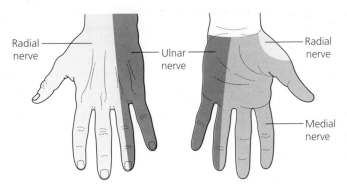

Figure 2.18 Sensory dermatomes

TONE

● Assess flexion and extension

MOTOR

Ask the patient to:

● Squeeze your fingers (C8/T1) and then spread their fingers (C7)
● Hold a piece of paper between the fingers: pull (dorsal abductors – ulnar)
● Push their thumbs to the ceiling (medial nerve)
● Oppose your pincer grip with theirs (opponens pollicis – medial)

Note:

● Medial nerve supplies 'LOAF' muscles: lumbricals, opponens pollicis, abductor pollicis brevis and flexor pollicis brevis
● Ulnar nerve supplies all the other small muscles of the hand, e.g. the interossei
● Radial nerve supplies the wrist extensors

FUNCTION

● Prayer and reverse prayer sign
● Turn in a light bulb/open a door handle
● Undo buttons, hold a pen/write, turn a key and pick up coins
● Ask about: combing hair, washing, dressing, teeth cleaning, opening jars

FURTHER TESTS

● X-ray relevant joints (± the ones above and below) and aspirate effusions in joints

OSTEOARTHRITIS

This common degenerative disease occurs predominantly in the older population. It is the commonest cause of arthritis and varies a great deal with respect to severity and restriction of function. Osteoarthritis most commonly affects the small joints of the hand, the spine, knees and hips, but can affect any joint in the body.

Table 2.4 Clinical features to differentiate osteoarthritis from rheumatoid arthritis

	Osteoarthritis	Rheumatoid arthritis
Joints	Asymmetrically affected	Symmetrically affected
	Distal small joints of hand	Proximal small joints of hand
		Erythema due to active inflammation
Deformity	Herberden's nodes	Boutonnière's
	Bouchard's nodes	Swan-neck
	Square thumbs	Z thumbs
Swelling	Bony, hard	Firm/spongy, warm
Nodules	Not present	Hand, tendons, elbow
Wasting	Present	Present
Movement	Restricted	Restricted
Stiffness	Worse with overuse	Morning stiffness significant

RISK FACTORS

- Previous trauma/repetitive occupational injury
- Concomitant inflammatory arthropathy, e.g. rheumatoid arthritis
- Past medical history, e.g. of haemochromatosis, acromegaly
- Obesity
- Age >45 years
- Family history

HISTORY

- Arthralgia (worsens with exertion)
- Minimal morning joint stiffness (<30 minutes)
- Joint deformity (see below)

INSPECTION

- Symmetry
- Deformity:
  - DIP joints – Heberden's nodes
  - PIP joints – Bouchard's nodes
  - Subluxation of thumb at first metacarpal – 'square thumb'
  - Genu varus or valgus
  - Pelvic tilt (positive Trendelenburg's test – see p. 111)
- Swelling: bony
- Muscle wasting, e.g. quadriceps (disuse)
- Scars: previous surgery, e.g. joint replacements, arthroscopy
- Skin changes:
  - Atrophy from repeated steroid injections
  - Erythema: bursitis/septic arthritis

PALPATION

- Crepitus
- Reduced range of movement, e.g. by pain

INVESTIGATIONS

- Blood tests to investigate for potential underlying causes if suggestive features in history/examination:
    - Rheumatoid arthritis (e.g. rheumatoid factor)
    - Haemochromatosis (e.g. iron studies)
    - Acromegaly (e.g. glucose tolerance test)
- X-ray of joints involved – typical features include:
    - Loss of joint space
    - Osteophytes
    - Osteosclerosis

Note: X-ray appearances do *not* necessarily correlate with clinical features

- MRI: provides more detailed imaging of joints

MANAGEMENT

Multidisciplinary team approach is key. This includes:

- Weight loss (diet and exercise advice)
- Physiotherapy
- Occupational therapy
- Walking aids (orthotics)
- Analgesia:
    - Paracetamol
    - NSAIDs/cyclo-oxygenase-2 (COX-2) inhibitors
    - Opiates
- Intra-articular steroid injections may be of some limited benefit
- Transcutaneous electrical nerve stimulation (TENS)
- Surgery
    - Joint arthroscopy
    - Osteotomy
    - Joint replacement

RHEUMATOID ARTHRITIS

This inflammatory arthritis is an autoimmune condition occurring predominantly in middle-aged females (female to male ratio 3:1), typically causing pain, erythema and swelling. It most commonly affects the small joints of the hands and feet, but can progress to other joints in the body. It also has several other manifestations (Box 2.59).

HISTORY

- Arthralgia (worsens with exertion)
- Morning joint stiffness (>30 minutes)
- Joint swelling and erythema
- Joint deformity (see below)
- Systemic symptoms, e.g. fatigue, malaise, loss of appetite/weight

> **BOX 2.59 EXTRA-ARTICULAR MANIFESTATIONS OF RHEUMATOID ARTHRITIS**
>
> Skin – nodules
> Haematological – anaemia, e.g. secondary to:
> - Anaemia of chronic disease
> - Felty's syndrome (see below)
> - Folic acid deficiency or secondary to disease-modifying antirheumatic drugs (DMARDs) – marrow suppression; NSAIDs – gastrointestinal bleeding
>
> Vasculitis – Raynaud's, leg ulcers, nail-fold infarcts
> Cardiac – pericarditis, conduction defects
> Neurological – cervical myelopathy, peripheral neuropathy, carpal tunnel syndrome
> Ophthalmic – episcleritis, Sjögren's syndrome
> Others – Felty's syndrome (rheumatoid arthritis with splenomegaly, haemolytic anaemia), pulmonary rheumatoid nodules
> Other autoimmune disease, e.g. pernicious anaemia, vitiligo

INSPECTION

General

- Low BMI
- Scars – from previous surgery
- Pallor – secondary to anaemia

Eyes

- Dry eyes (Sjögren's)
- Scleritis/episcleritis

Hands

- Nail-fold infarcts
- Palmar erythema
- Symmetrical deforming arthropathy affecting proximal small joints of hands and feet (Box 2.60)
- Muscle wasting
- Small joint swelling
- Psoriatic rash
- Rheumatoid nodules, e.g. over tendons

Other joints

Assess other joints for signs of arthropathy, e.g. swelling, deformity. Rheumatoid arthritis also affects:

- Feet
- Ankles
- Knees, hips
- Spine – especially atlanto-axial joint (subluxation)

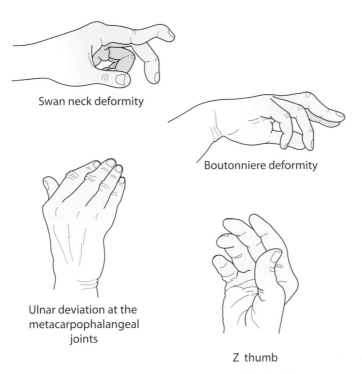

Swan neck deformity

Boutonniere deformity

Ulnar deviation at the
metacarpophalangeal
joints

Z thumb

Figure 2.19 Common deformities in rheumatoid arthritis

BOX 2.60 SMALL JOINT DEFORMITY OF RA

- Swan-neck – hyperextension of PIP, fixed flexion of the DIP and MCP joints
- Boutonnière's – fixed flexion of PIP joints, extension of DIP and MCP joints
- 'Z' thumb
- Ulnar deviation – subluxation of the MCP joints

PALPATION

- Reduced range of movement, e.g. secondary to pain
- Joint subluxation/dislocation

INVESTIGATIONS

- Blood tests
  - ○ FBC, e.g. haemoglobin for anaemia
  - ○ Full autoantibody screen
  - ○ Iron studies to exclude haemochromatosis
- X-ray of joints involved – typical features include:
  - ○ Loss of joint space
  - ○ Erosions
  - ○ Osteophytes
  - ○ Osteosclerosis

Note: X-ray appearances do *not* necessarily correlate with clinical features

- MRI: provides more detailed imaging of joints

MANAGEMENT

Many patients employ a combination of the therapies below to control their symptoms and delay disease progression. They include:

- Physiotherapy
- Occupational therapy
- Walking aids (orthotics)
- Complementary therapies, e.g. acupuncture, hydrotherapy
- Analgesia:
  - Paracetamol
  - NSAIDs/COX-2 inhibitors
  - Opiates
  - Neuromodulators
- DMARDs:
  - Include methotrexate, gold, penicillamine
  - Potentially toxic side effects include: pulmonary fibrosis, bone marrow suppression, renal failure, liver failure
  - Good evidence for therapeutic benefit
- Steroids:
  - Systemic – pulsed, continuous
  - Intra-articular injections
- Biological therapies, e.g. Anti tumour necrosis factor (TNF) α for those in whom conventional treatment fails
- Surgery, e.g. joint replacement

PSORIATIC ARTHRITIS

There are five types of psoriatic arthritis, some of which may resemble clinical features of RA.

They all exhibit the classical features of psoriatic skin changes (see p. 159), especially dorsal surface of the hands feet and over the elbows as well as nail pitting. Remember though the area of skin affected by psoriasis may be very small and even hidden, e.g. under hair.

- Symmetrical – rheumatoid-like joint involvement but milder disease course
- Asymmetrical – similar distribution of joints to osteoarthritis but redness and tenderness are present, with sausage digits
- Spondylitis – affecting spine, similar to ankylosing spondylitis
- Arthritis mutilans – destructive, severe form affecting small joints of hands and feet (e.g. telescopic digits)
- DIP type – similar to osteoarthritis but showing preference for these hand joints

CARPAL TUNNEL SYNDROME

This common condition presents in the middle aged and may be a manifestation of many underlying medical conditions. It arises as a result of compression of the median nerve as it passes through the carpal tunnel of the wrist.

HISTORY

- Patient complains of numbness or tingling in hand and arm
- Worse at night
- Relieved by dangling hand over bed
- May be bilateral

BOX 2.61 CAUSES OF CARPAL TUNNEL SYNDROME

- Idiopathic
- Hypothyroidism
- Repetitive use
- Rheumatoid arthritis
- Pregnancy
- Osteoarthritis

- Obesity
- Amyloidosis (primary)
- Acromegaly
- Oral contraceptive
- Diabetes
- Gout

INTRODUCTION

- Introduce yourself to the patient
- Explain the procedure and gain consent
- Ask about pain
- Expose to above the elbows
- Place forearms/hands on a pillow
- Ensure lighting is adequate

INSPECTION

General

- Commonly:
  - Middle aged
  - Female
- Pregnant
- Obvious medical disease
  - Acromegaly: characteristic appearance
  - Thyroid disease: appearance, scars
  - Rheumatoid arthritis

Hands

- Look for:
  - Wasting of thenar eminence
- Power:
  - Weakness in thumb opposition, abduction and flexion
- Sensation:
  - Reduced sensation or tingling over palmar thumb, first, middle and index finger

BOX 2.62 MEDIAN NERVE

- Roots: C6-T1
- Sensory distribution: palmar area of lateral hand, index, middle and other half of ring finger
- Motor supply to: 'LOAF' muscles: lumbricals, opponens pollicis, abductor pollicis brevis and flexor pollicis brevis

INVESTIGATIONS

- Tinel's sign: percussion over the carpal tunnels reproduces symptoms
- Phalen's sign: flexion of both wrists whilst putting pressure over the carpal tunnels for 60 seconds reproduces symptoms
- Nerve conduction studies (most reliable test)

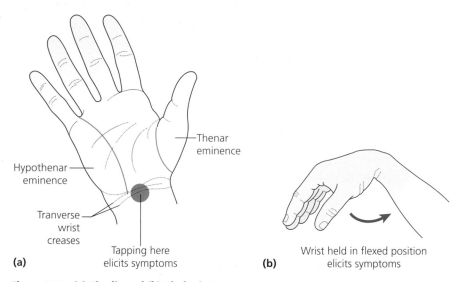

Figure 2.20 (a) Tinel's and (b) Phalen's tests.

TREATMENT

- Conservative: hand splints
- Medical: steroid injection
- Surgery: decompression

SYSTEMIC LUPUS ERYTHEMATOSUS

Systemic lupus erythematosus is a multisystem autoimmune disease with numerous manifestations. It commonly presents in young to middle-aged females (9:1 female to male ratio).

INSPECTION

- General:
  - Young female patient
  - Myalgia/polymyositis
  - Ankle oedema – nephrotic syndrome
- Skin:
  - Livedo reticularis – 'crazy-paving' rash
  - Vasculitis
  - Scarring alopecia
- Hands:
  - Arthritis (non-erosive)
  - Raynaud's syndrome
- Face:
  - Bilateral erythematous butterfly (malar) rash:
    - Located on cheeks, nose, chin and other sun-exposed areas of the body
    - Typically spares the nasolabial folds
    - Associated with plugged follicles, scaling and scarring
  - Mouth ulcers (painless)
- Eyes:
  - Sjögren's syndrome
  - Papilloedema
  - Haemorrhages and white exudates
- Heart:
  - Endocarditis murmur – Libman–Sachs (non-infective) endocarditis
  - Myocarditis
  - Pericardial rub
  - Pericardial effusion
- Lungs:
  - Pleural effusion
  - Pulmonary fibrosis (rare)
- Abdomen:
  - Hepatomegaly
  - Renal disease – proteinuria, haematuria
- Nervous system:
  - Peripheral neuropathy
  - Mononeuritis multiplex
  - Psychiatric disease

> ### BOX 2.63 AMERICAN COLLEGE OF RHEUMATOLOGY CRITERIA FOR THE DIAGNOSIS OF SYSTEMIC LUPUS ERYTHEMATOSUS
>
> (Need 4 out of 11 of which only one is a skin manifestation)
>
> - Malar rash
> - Photosensitive rash
> - Discoid rash
> - Serositis (peritonitis, pericardial, pleural)
> - Arthritis (more than two joints)
> - Mucositis (mouth and nasopharyngeal ulcers)
> - Renal disease
> - CNS disease (seizures, psychosis)
> - Haematological – low platelets, low white cells, autoimmune haemolytic anaemia
> - Antinuclear antibody positive
> - Other antibody positivity, e.g. anti-dsDNA, anti-Sm

ASSOCIATIONS

- Discoid lupus
- Drug-induced lupus
  - More common in males
  - Does not affect kidneys or CNS, but more commonly the lungs
  - Resolves on stopping responsible drug, e.g. penicillamine, phenytoin, oral contraceptive
  - Anti-dsDNA autoantibodies negative
- Antiphospholipid syndrome

TREATMENT

- Skin – sunblock/avoid exposure
- NSAIDs/antimalarial drugs for arthritis
- Steroids/immunosuppressants for nephritis

SYSTEMIC SCLEROSIS

Systemic sclerosis is a multisystem connective tissue disease that causes widespread fibrosis. It can be localized or systemic. The latter can be subdivided into diffuse or limited.

- Localized scleroderma – patients develop isolated areas of skin sclerosis such as morphoea (indurated, violaceous plaques) and 'coup de sabre' linear sclerosis
- Limited and diffuse systemic sclerosis – both affect numerous organ systems but are differentiated according to their degree of skin involvement

LIMITED ('CREST') SYSTEMIC SCLEROSIS

- Skin disease is limited to the hands, forearms, feet, neck and face
- Patients may report dysphagia and painful digits, especially when cold
- Other manifestations include:
  - **C**alcinosis – tender, hard calcium deposits, e.g. on the fingers
  - **R**aynaud's phenomenon – common, causes hands to go painfully white, blue then red, when cold

- ○   (**E**) oEsophageal dysmotility – frequently causes dysphagia
  - ○   **S**clerodactyly – skin is tight, shiny and painful over digits
  - ○   **T**elangiectasia – commonly over the face and chest
- Some features of the diffuse form may also be present and vice versa

DIFFUSE SYSTEMIC SCLEROSIS

- Skin disease is more widespread affecting chest, trunk and proximal limbs
- Organ involvement is more widespread and in addition to 'CREST' symptoms and signs patients may have:
  - ○   Pulmonary fibrosis
  - ○   Pulmonary hypertension (although more common in limited form)
  - ○   Cardiac involvement, e.g. conduction defects, pericardial fibrosis
  - ○   Renal failure (more common in diffuse form)
  - ○   Peripheral vascular disease, e.g. ulceration
  - ○   Polyarthritis and contractures

EXAMINATION

A multisystem examination is warranted, including:

- Cardiac: arrhythmias, pericardial effusion, pulmonary hypertension, cor pulmonale, poor/absent peripheral pulses
- Respiratory: dyspnoea, bilateral crackles
- Hands: shiny tight skin over digits, calcinosis nodules, telangiectasia, atrophic nails, Raynaud's phenomenon
- Face: shiny, tight skin causing microstomia (small mouth) and 'beak-like' nose, multiple telangiectasia
- Joints: inflammatory arthritis
- Related diseases, i.e. autoimmune diseases – vitiligo, primary biliary cirrhosis

INVESTIGATIONS

- Antinuclear antibodies (positive >95 per cent cases)
  - ○   Anticentromere autoantibodies (fewer than half of patients with limited disease)
  - ○   Antitopoisomerase (half of patients with diffuse disease)
  - ○   Antinucleolar antibodies (fewer than half of patients with diffuse disease)
- ECG – arrhythmias, conduction defects
- Echocardiogram – to assess fibrosis, effusions
- Thoracic high-resolution CT – to assess pulmonary fibrosis
- Pulmonary function tests
- Biopsy and histological examination if diagnosis unclear

TREATMENT

There is no effective treatment to reverse disease progression. Symptomatic and supportive treatment is therefore key:

- DMARDs may have an unproven role in treating skin disease
- Raynaud's: keep hands warm, vasodilators, intravenous prostacyclin
- Pulmonary fibrosis may respond to immunosuppressants such as cyclophosphamide

- Renal decline may be slowed with ACE inhibitors
- Joint disease may respond to conventional analgesia
- Occupational therapists can help manage disability thereby increasing functional abilities

SARCOIDOSIS

This is a multisystem disease characterized by non-caseating granulomas, predominantly affecting the lungs, brain, eyes, kidneys, liver and skin. It is more common in Afro-Caribbean females.

HISTORY
General

- Often asymptomatic
- Lethargy malaise
- Weight loss
- Fever, night sweats

Organ-specific

- Arthralgia
- Rash, skin changes
- Dry cough, shortness of breath
- Painful, erythematous eyes
- Parotitis
- Weakness, numbness

EXAMINATION
General

- Low BMI

Skin

- Erythema nodosum – tender nodules on anterior shins
- Lupus pernio – violaceous rash over cheeks, nose and chin

Musculoskeletal

- Polyarthritis
- Myositis

Eyes

- Uveitis
- Conjunctivitis

Respiratory

- Non-productive cough
- Dyspnoea
- Rarely effusions and haemoptysis

Neurology

Owing to its wide distribution sarcoidosis can produce a variety of central and peripheral, UMN and LMN neurological symptoms and signs. Common manifestations include:

- Facial nerve palsy
- Peripheral neuropathy (see p. 80)

Cardiac

- Conduction defects
- Peri- or myocarditis
- Cor pulmonale

Renal

- Stones
- Renal failure

Liver

- Portal hypertension
- Hepatomegaly

INVESTIGATIONS

- Blood tests:
  - FBC: raised white cells, eosinophilia
  - ESR – raised
  - Renal function
  - Bone profile – hypercalcaemia (due to excessive vitamin D activation by granulomas), raised phosphate
  - LFTs – raised alkaline phosphatase
  - Serum angiotensin-converting enzyme level – raised in >70 per cent cases
  - Thyroid function (sarcoid is often associated with thyroid disease)
  - Falsely raised autoantibodies, e.g. rheumatoid factor, antinuclear antibodies
- 24-hour urine calcium (increased)
- ECG
- Chest X-ray: classically bilateral hilar lymphadenopathy, pulmonary infiltrates
- Pulmonary function tests: often exhibit a restrictive pattern
- Ophthalmology review

TREATMENT

- Observation, i.e. no treatment required owing to spontaneous remission (>50 per cent recover within 3 years)
- Systemic steroids
- Steroid-sparing agents, e.g. methotrexate

ANKYLOSING SPONDYLITIS

This progressive seronegative arthropathy predominantly affects the axial skeleton, but also exhibits several important extra-articular manifestations. It is commonly encountered in

OSCE stations when examining the spine as the clinical picture is characteristic of the disease.

INTRODUCTION

- Introduce yourself, explain procedure and request permission
- Enquire about any pain or discomfort
- Ensure adequate lighting
- Ask the patient to remove their clothes to their underwear

INSPECTION

Spine

- Loss of lumbar lordosis
- Extension of the cervical spine
- Stooped 'question mark' posture
- Fixed kyphosis
- Restricted spinal movement in all directions: patient moves '*en bloc*'

Others

- Reduced chest expansion
- Prominent abdomen
- Coexisting psoriatic arthritis

Eyes

- Anterior uveitis/iritis

EXAMINATION

Spine

- Modified Schober's test

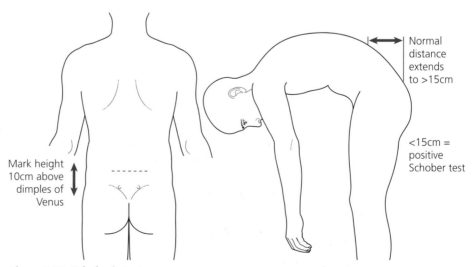

Normal distance extends to >15cm

<15cm = positive Schober test

Mark height 10cm above dimples of Venus

Figure 2.21 Schober's test

- While the patient is standing, mark a distance of 10 cm above the sacral dimples, on their back
- Ask them to attempt to touch their toes
- The normal distance expands from 10 cm to 15 cm (dimples to line)
- Patients with ankylosing spondylitis will exhibit restricted lumbar flexion (positive test)
- Wall occiput test
    - Ask the patient to stand with their back and heels against a wall
    - Ask them to place their occiput against the wall at the same time
    - Patients with ankylosing spondylitis will be unable to touch the wall with their head

Cardiovascular system

- Examine for aortic regurgitation

Respiratory

- Examine for apical pulmonary fibrosis

Feet

- Examine the sole of the feet for a thickened, painful plantar fascia indicating plantar fasciitis

Assess function

- Enquire about the patient's ability to perform day to day activities, e.g.:
    - Washing and dressing
    - Cooking and shopping
    - Driving

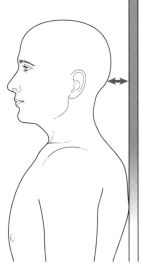

Figure 2.22 Wall occiput test

BOX 2.64 'As' ASSOCIATED WITH ANKYLOSING SPONDYLITIS

- Atrioventricular conduction block
- Aortic regurgitation and aortitis
- Apical lung fibrosis
- Amyloidosis
- Anterior uveitis
- Achilles tendonitis

INVESTIGATIONS

- Blood tests:
    - Human leucocyte antigen (HLA)-B27 positive
    - C-reactive protein (CRP), ESR – raised in active disease
- ECG:
    - Atrioventricular heart block
- Imaging:
- X-rays of the axial spine may show:
    - Sacroiliitis
    - Bamboo spine
    - Loss of lumbar lordosis

Note: X-ray changes are often normal in active disease.

- Ophthalmology referral – if evidence of eye disease
- Pulmonary function tests – if evidence of lung fibrosis, reduced chest expansion

TREATMENT

- Physiotherapy
- Simple analgesia, e.g. NSAIDs
- DMARDs
- Anti-TNF agents are being used increasingly in severe disease

GOUT

Gout is caused by accumulation of uric acid crystals in the joints and soft tissues. There are two main types: acute mono-articular attacks and chronic tophaceous gout.

BOX 2.65 CAUSES OF GOUT

Drugs:
- Aspirin
- Diuretics

Increased purine intake:
- Diet
- Alcohol excess

Increased purine production:
- Inborn errors of metabolism
- Increased cell lysis, e.g. lymphoproliferative disease, tumour lysis syndrome

Decreased purine/urate excretion:
- Renal failure

EXAMINATION

- Joint(s):
  - Red, hot
  - Swollen
  - Tender
  - Gouty tophi
  - Unilateral/asymmetrical distribution (the hallux is a classical site for attacks of gout)
- Ear:
  - Gouty tophi

INVESTIGATIONS

- Routine blood tests including:
  - Uric acid level (may be normal)
  - Renal function
- Synovial fluid aspiration:
  - High white cell count
  - Intra- and extracellular needle-shaped *negatively* birefringent crystals
- Joint X-rays:
  - No/minimal changes
  - Late features include erosions, sclerosis, calcified gouty tophi

TREATMENT
Pain control

- ○ NSAIDs
- ○ Colchicine (if NSAIDs contraindicated)
- ○ Oral steroids (less commonly used)

Prophylaxis

- Allopurinol prophylaxis if experiencing recurrent bouts – this must not be started during an attack as it will worsen symptoms acutely

PSEUDOGOUT

- This is also known as calcium pyrophosphate deposition disease and is similar in presentation and treatment to gout. There is no agent available for prophylaxis
- Synovial fluid analysis may however show rhomboid crystals that are *positively* birefringent under polarized light

SURGERY

LUMPS AND BUMPS

INTRODUCTION

- Introduce yourself to the patient
- Explain the examination and gain consent
- Explain the examination
- Ask if painful
- Request permission
- Expose appropriately

INSPECTION

- Site
- Shape: spherical, elliptical, flat, raised
- Size: measure in centimetres
- Number: solitary, multiple
- Margin: raised/flat, well/ill-defined, irregular/smooth
- Surface: smooth, irregular, ulcerated, bleeding
- Colour: light/dark/mixed, red
- Associated skin changes: scaling, erythema (see p. 157)

EXAMINATION

- Tenderness
- Temperature
- Consistency: soft, firm, hard
- Fluctuance: cystic, solid
- Fixation: mobile, deep/superficial tethering
- Transillumination

- Pulsatile: if so
  - ○ Auscultate for thrill
  - ○ Compressible (venous aneurysm)
- If hernia suspected (see p. 66):
  - ○ Cough impulse
  - ○ Reducibility
- Request to assess regional lymph nodes

Table 2.5 Common lesions

Lesion	Site	Description
Sebaceous cyst	Scalp, face, neck, back	Smooth, spherical, soft/firm, immobile; punctum characteristic
Lipoma	Trunk, shoulders, neck, axilla	Smooth, soft, mobile, within subcutaneous tissue, occasionally intramuscular with tethering to muscle
Ganglion	Dorsum of hand, wrist, ankle	Smooth, spherical, firm, fluctuant, immobile
Lymph node	Groin, neck, axilla	Malignant: hard, non-tender, tethered, solitary Inflammatory: firm, tender, mobile, multiple
Melanoma	Anywhere	Irregular edge and pigmentation, ulceration/bleeding, flat/raised
Basal cell carcinoma (rodent ulcer)	Sun exposed areas 'Mask area'	Firm pearly nodule with surface telangiectasia, or ulcer with rolled edges, local invasion is destructive
Squamous cell carcinoma	Sun exposed areas, lips	Ulcer with hard raised edges

INVESTIGATIONS

- Lesions where the diagnosis of a benign lesion is not clear are investigated by excision
- For subcutaneous lesions that have suspicious features such as tethering, pain, or recurrence then ultrasound or MRI can help exclude sinister features prior to excision
- Suspected soft tissue sarcomas *must not* be investigated with biopsy or fine-needle aspiration but wide excision due to the potential seeding of tumour cells

TREATMENT

- Indication for excision:
  - ○ Patient wishes/worries
  - ○ Pain
  - ○ Increase in size
  - ○ Repeated infections
  - ○ Itching
  - ○ Bleeding
- Skin lesions:
  - ○ Small lesions: excision
  - ○ Large lesions: especially malignancy, may require skin grafting
- Subcutaneous lesions:
  - ○ Simple lipomas sometimes require excision to reassure the patient. A very small proportion can progress to malignant liposarcomas
  - ○ Sebaceous cysts can be monitored but require excision if there is an episode of infection or change in size

VASCULAR EXAMINATION

INTRODUCTION

- Explain the examination
- Ask about painful areas
- Request permission
- Position patient lying flat with arms by their sides and head rested
- Expose appropriately (e.g. lower limbs and feet)

INSPECTION

General

- Pallor
- Central cyanosis
- Previous scars
- Xanthelasma
- Corneal arcus

Hands

- Peripheral cyanosis
- Splinter haemorrhages
- Tar staining

Limbs

- Scars (from previous surgery)
- Muscle wasting, asymmetry
- Oedema
- Skin colour: red, white, purple, blue
- Trophic changes:
  - Shiny skin
  - Hair loss
  - Loss of subcutaneous tissue

Pressure points

- Lateral foot
- First metatarsal
- Heel
- Malleoli
- Toes

Ulcers

- Position
- Size
- Shape
- Depth
- Edge character
- Base colour, contents

PALPATION

- Temperature: cool suggests poor circulation, compare with other side
- Pitting oedema: tested for independent locations: dorsum of foot/shin/sacrum
- Pulses:
  - Radial: rate/rhythm
  - Brachial pulse and blood pressure
  - Femoral: mid-inguinal point
  - Popliteal: 30° knee flexion – press firmly with both hands: thumbs in front and four fingers behind knee – aneurysmal if easily palpable
  - Posterior tibial (PT): below and behind medial malleolus
  - Dorsalis pedis (DP): middle of dorsum of foot just lateral to extensor hallucis

AUSCULTATION

- Femoral/carotid bruits

ADDITIONAL TESTS

- Buerger's test
  - Note supine colour of soles (should be pink)
  - Elevate leg to 45°: ideally two legs at once for >1 min then lower to dependent position (i.e. below the bed)
  - If they go pale on elevation with reactive hyperaemia on dependency, the test is positive and ischaemia should be suspected
- Ankle–brachial pressure index (ABPI)
  - Calculated by dividing the highest systolic blood pressure in the arteries at the ankle (PT) and foot (DP) by the higher of the two systolic blood pressures in the arms
  - 1= normal, 0.5–0.8 occlusion, <0.5 critical ischaemia
  - Care is needed in diabetes where calcification of vessels may give falsely high readings

COMPLETE EXAMINATION

Examine the abdomen for AAAs and radio-femoral delay.

BOX 2.66 ACUTELY ISCHAEMIC LEG: THE SIX Ps

- Pain
- Pallor
- Pulselessness
- Perishing cold
- Paralysis (poor prognosis)
- Paraesthesiae (poor prognosis)

This is a surgical emergency: revascularize within 4–6 hours

BREAST EXAMINATION

INTRODUCTION

- Ensure a chaperone is present and ensure privacy
- Explain the examination and request permission
- Ask about painful areas/lumps
- Position patient at 45°
- Expose appropriately (expose to waist)

INSPECTION

- Look for asymmetry with arms above head and then on hips
- Note any:
  - Peau d'orange (dimpled skin)
  - Puckering
  - Nipple inversion or discharge
  - Skin changes/eczema
  - Obvious lumps
  - Colour change

BOX 2.67 DIFFERENTIAL DIAGNOSIS OF BREAST LUMPS

Benign:
- Lipoma
- Sebaceous cyst
- Fibroadenoma
- Fat necrosis
- Abscess

Malignant:
- Carcinoma
- Phyllodes tumour

PALPATION

- Ensure patient at 45° with arms above head and as relaxed as possible
- Ask if any areas are painful and to point to any lumps
- Start with normal breast:
  - Using flat of hand either spirally outwards or over four quadrants
  - Pay particular attention to areola – pressing onto chest wall to flatten it out

If you feel a lump

Complete breast examination on that side then return to lump and note:

- Size
- Shape
- Consistency (soft/firm/hard)
- Skin changes
- Tethering

> **BOX 2.68 ASSESSING LUMP FIXATION**
>
> - Palpate lump between thumb and forefinger – skin tethered lump will move with skin.
> - Ask the patient to push her hand down into her hips – a muscle tethered lump will now remain static on underlying pectoral muscle

Axilla

- Hold left hand in your left hand and vice versa taking weight of arm
- Palpate medially, laterally, posteriorly, anteriorly, apically

Regional lymph nodes

- Palpate supraclavicular fossa paying particular attention to Virchow's node
- Palpate infraclavicular nodes

Complete examination

Ask to:

- Palpate neck lymph nodes
- Palpate liver for metastases (nodular edge/enlarged)
- Percuss posterior chest for metastases and lung bases for effusion

FURTHER INVESTIGATIONS

Triple assessment:

- History and examination
- Histology: fine needle aspiration/core biopsy
- Radiology: mammography/ultrasound

VARICOSE VEINS EXAMINATION

INTRODUCTION

- Explain the examination
- Ask about painful areas
- Request permission
- Position patient standing
- Expose both limbs from groin to foot

INSPECTION

- Ankle oedema ('beer bottle shape')
- Large visible veins
  - Site
  - Distribution:
    - long saphenous vein: medial thigh, anteromedial shin
    - short saphenous vein: posterior calf

- Skin (especially in the 'gaiter region')
  - Ulcers (above medial malleolus)
  - Haemosiderin deposits
  - Eczema
  - Thin skin
  - Oedema
  - Venous stars
  - Lipodermatosclerosis
- Scars: in groin, along long saphenous veins – small avulsion scars (previous surgery)

PALPATION

- Assess for pitting oedema
- Lipodermatosclerosis (thick, fibrotic skin)
- Temperature (compare the legs with back of hand)
- Saphenofemoral junction (SFJ; 3 cm below and lateral to the pubic tubercle) for:
  - Saphena varix (feels like an underfilled balloon that empties with pressure)
  - Cough impulse (implies incompetence at SFJ)

TESTS

(These are time consuming so offer them to the examiner prior to proceeding.)

- Doppler scan – nowadays assessment of varicose veins is invariably performed by Doppler ultrasound scan and colour duplex studies
- Tap test:
  - Place fingers of one hand at lower limit of a long varicose vein
  - Tap at upper limit with other hand
  - Percussion impulse indicates incompetent intervening valves
- Trendelenburg's test:
  - Determines SFJ incompetence (positive if incompetent)
  - Lie patient flat and elevate leg until veins emptied
  - Place two fingers over SFJ and ask patient to stand, keeping fingers in place:
    - If varicosities fill – communicating valves are incompetent
    - If no filling but veins fill on release of fingers – SFJ is incompetent
- Tourniquet test (if Trendelenburg's test does not reveal incompetent SFJ):
  - Defines segment containing incompetent perforators
  - Lie patient flat and elevate leg
  - Place rubber tourniquet around mid-thigh and stand patient up
  - If:
    - The veins above the tourniquet fill, those below stay collapsed the incompetent communicating vein is above the tourniquet
    - The veins fill below the tourniquet, the incompetent communicating vein/perforators are below the tourniquet
  - Repeat down the leg between site of perforators until veins below stay collapsed – this defines the segment containing incompetent perforators
- Perthes' test:
  - Place tourniquet at SFJ around the elevated leg so veins below are empty
  - Ask patient to stand up and down on tip-toe 10 times
  - Filling of superficial veins and pain in legs indicates deep venous occlusion

AUSCULTATION

- Listen for bruits over sites of marked venous clusters

COMPLETE EXAMINATION

- Offer to examine:
  - Abdomen (for masses that could cause intravenous obstruction, e.g. pregnancy)
  - Rectum
  - Pelvis in females/external genitalia in men

BOX 2.69 SURFACE ANATOMY AT THE ANKLE

- Long saphenous vein – anterior to medial malleolus
- Short saphenous vein – behind lateral malleolus

ULCERS

INTRODUCTION

- Explain the examination
- Ask if painful
- Request permission
- Position patient at 45°
- Expose appropriately (lower limb and foot)

INSPECTION

- Site:
  - Tuberculosis: neck, groin, axilla
  - Malignancy: anywhere

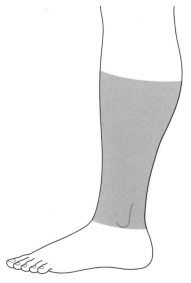

Figure 2.23 'Gaiter' distribution of venous ulceration

- ○ Vascular: lower limb
  - ◆ Between toes, pressure areas (diabetic, neuropathic ulcers)
  - ◆ Extremities (ischaemic ulcers)
  - ◆ Gaiter area: above malleoli, especially medial (venous ulcers)
- Measure:
  - ○ Size
  - ○ Depth
- Base:
  - ○ Healing: red, granulation tissue
  - ○ Ischaemic: black eschar
  - ○ Basal cell carcinoma (BCC): 'pearly'
  - ○ Neuropathic, ischaemic: tendon, bone exposed
- Discharge:
  - ○ Infective: purulent, offensive odour
  - ○ Granulation or malignancy: bleeding
- Temperature:
  - ○ Neuropathic, infected: hot
  - ○ Ischaemic: cold
- Edge:
  - ○ Flat/sloping (traumatic/venous)
  - ○ Punched out (ischaemic, neuropathic, tertiary syphilis)
  - ○ Raised (BCC)
  - ○ Raised and everted, i.e. rolled (squamous cell carcinoma [SCC])
- Sensation:
  - ○ Painful (ischaemic, venous)
  - ○ Painless (diabetic, neuropathic)
- To complete examination:
  - ○ Palpate any regional lymph nodes (secondary infection, malignant spread)
  - ○ Neurological examination: sensation and power (diabetic/neuropathic)
  - ○ Examine for varicose veins (venous)
  - ○ Complete a vascular examination, e.g. peripheral pulses (ischaemic)

INVESTIGATIONS

- Histological examination
- Cytological examination: biopsy, scrapings
- Microbiology: swabs, scrapings for microscopy, culture and sensitivities

---

BOX 2.70 FEATURES OF COMMON ULCERS

Venous:
- Gaiter area
- Sloping edge
- Associated varicose veins
- Chronic venous hypertension: eczema, lipodermatosclerosis, haemosiderosis
- Marjolin's ulcer: malignant change within chronic venous ulcer

Ischaemic:
- Extremities

- Punched out
- Necrotic skin
- Chronic ischaemic changes: hairless, cold, pulseless

Diabetic:
- Pressure areas
- Painless
- Punched out
- Infection: plantar abscesses, osteomyelitis
- Charcot joints

ENDOCRINE

NECK EXAMINATION

INTRODUCTION

- Explain the examination
- Ask about painful areas
- Request permission
- Position patient in chair or on a couch, which you can get behind
- Expose neck appropriately

INSPECTION

Generally

- Signs of thyroid disease, e.g.:
  - Dress – appropriate for time of year
  - Pulse – tachycardic or bradycardic
  - Tremor
  - Eye signs: exophthalmos, lid lag, chemosis
  - Hypothyroid 'facies' – dry skin, coarse features
  - Thinning hair
  - Pretibial myxoedema
- Superior vena cava obstruction:
  - Plethora
  - Raised JVP
  - Distended veins on upper thorax

Neck

- Swelling, obvious goitre
- Thyroidectomy scar

- Whilst visualizing the neck, ask the patient to take a sip of water in their mouth
  - Ask them to swallow the water while observing the movement of any thyroid masses
  - Ask the patient to put out their tongue (thyroglossal cyst will move superiorly)

PALPATION

- Start from standing behind patient
- Warn them it may feel slightly uncomfortable
- Using your index and middle fingers from both hands gently palpate the thyroid
- Ask the patient to protrude tongue and note any movement in the thyroid
- Ask the patient to take a sip of water in their mouth, hold it and swallow whilst palpating again for any movement
- Note the features of any mass:
  - Size
  - Shape
  - Consistency
  - Diffuse or nodular
  - Fixation
- Go on to examine the cervical lymph nodes (see p. 64)
- Look for any tracheal deviation
- While standing behind look over the top of the head for exophthalmos

PERCUSSION

- Percuss over the sternum to elicit any retrosternal swelling

AUSCULTATION

- Listen over a thyroid mass for a bruit

OTHER SYSTEMS

- Lid lag: ask the patient to follow your finger vertically up and down (hyperthyroidism)
- Reflexes: look for slow relaxing reflexes (hypothyroidism)
- Proximal myopathy: ask them to rise from sitting without using their hands for support

ASK

- Do they feel warm or cold?
- Have they had any disruption of their bowel habit or appetite?
- Have they had any irregularity of their menstrual cycle?

FURTHER INVESTIGATIONS

- Thyroid function tests
- Thyroid autoantibodies
- Ultrasound scan neck

See pages 148 and 149.

HYPERTHYROIDISM

INTRODUCTION

- Ask permission
- Enquire about any pain or discomfort
- Ensure adequate lighting
- Expose the patient appropriately

INSPECTION

General

- Anxious, fidgety patient
- Thin
- Fine hair/receding hairline in females
- Febrile

Hands

- Warm
- Sweaty
- Tremulous (may be fine)
- Heart rate: tachycardia (sinus or atrial fibrillation)
- Thyroid acropachy (looks like clubbing)
- Onycholysis (often bilaterally on fourth finger)

Neck

- As for neck examination (see p. 146)
- May or may not have diffuse or nodular goitre, with an overlying bruit (bilateral bruit specific to Graves' disease)
- Look for thyroidectomy scar

BOX 2.71 CAUSES OF HYPERTHYROIDISM

- Graves' disease – autoimmune disease, thyroid-stimulating hormone (TSH) receptor stimulating autoantibodies
- Toxic multinodular goitre or solitary nodule
- Post-partum thyroiditis – usually occurring between 2 and 10 months post-partum
- De Quervain's thyroiditis – caused by viral infection with fever and painful goitre
- Excess levothyroxine administration

Eyes

- Non-Graves' manifestations: lid retraction (upper sclera visible between cornea and lid) and lag, proptosis
- Graves' specific: exophthalmos (lower sclera visible between cornea and lower lid) and ophthalmoplegia

(**Note**: these patients are at risk from exposure keratitis.)

Cardiovascular system
- Tachycardia – sinus or atrial fibrillation
- Hypertension
- Systolic flow murmur
- High output cardiac failure

Legs
- Pretibial myxoedema – this only occurs in Graves' disease (bilateral, symmetrical, well defined lesions, red/brown, on shins and arms)
- Proximal muscle weakness
- Hyperreflexia

ASSOCIATED DISEASES

- Other autoimmune diseases – diabetes, Addison's, primary biliary cirrhosis

FURTHER INVESTIGATIONS

- Thyroid function tests
- Thyroid autoantibodies
- Ultrasound scan (neck)

TREATMENT

- Drugs:
  - β-Blockers, e.g. propranolol
  - Carbimazole
  - Propylthiouracil (preferred in pregnancy)
- Radiation: radioactive iodine
- Surgery: subtotal thyroidectomy
- Referral: ophthalmologist to assess eye disease

Note: If rendered hypothyroid by therapy, levothyroxine replacement treatment may be required

HYPOTHYROIDISM

INTRODUCTION

- Ask permission
- Enquire about any pain or discomfort
- Ensure adequate lighting
- Expose the patient appropriately

INSPECTION
General

- Overweight
- Non-pitting swelling throughout
- Signs of other autoimmune diseases, e.g. vitiligo, Addison's disease

Face

- 'Coarse' myxoedematous facies
- Thin, dry brittle hair
- Periorbital swelling
- Loss of outer third of the eyebrows

Hands

- Dry, thick skin
- Slow pulse

Neck

- As for neck examination (see p. 146)
- May or may not have diffuse goitre
- Look for a thyroidectomy scar

BOX 2.72 CAUSES OF HYPOTHYROIDISM

- Post radioactive iodine therapy or thyroidectomy
- Atrophic hypothyroidism
- Hashimoto's disease – autoimmune disease ± goitre
- De Quervain's thyroiditis – caused by viral infection with fever and painful goitre
- Pituitary disease
- Iodine deficiency (rare in developed countries)
- Congenital (rare)

Eyes

- Exophthalmos (with previously treated Graves' disease)

Cardiovascular system

- Bradycardia
- Hypertension

Legs

- Myopathy
- Slow relaxing reflexes

ASSOCIATED DISEASES

- Other autoimmune diseases – diabetes, Addison's disease, primary biliary cirrhosis, rheumatoid arthritis, pernicious anaemia
- Hypertension
- Dyslipidaemia
- Cardiovascular disease
- Carpal tunnel syndrome
- Anaemia

FURTHER INVESTIGATIONS

- Thyroid function tests
- Thyroid autoantibodies
- Ultrasound scan (neck)

TREATMENT

- Patients <60 years with no cardiovascular disease: approximately 50–100 µg levothyroxine daily
- Patients at high risk of cardiovascular disease: 25 µg daily and titrate up

CUSHING'S SYNDROME

This syndrome arises from corticosteroid excess due to a number of causes.

It should not be confused with Cushing's disease which occurs when the syndrome is caused by either an ACTH-secreting pituitary microadenoma or ectopic ACTH production from a malignancy.

INSPECTION
General

- 'Moon face'
- Supraclavicular fat pads
- 'Buffalo hump' interscapular fat pad
- Centripetal obesity
- Proximal muscle weakness

Skin

- Hirsutism
- Acne
- Purple striae
- Thin skin
- Poor wound healing
- Easy bruising
- Pigmentation (Cushing's disease)

Underlying disease

- Some diseases predispose to Cushing's syndrome as they often require long-term steroid therapy:
  - Renal transplant (e.g. fistula, scars, obvious transplanted kidney)
  - Asthma (inhaler, barrel chest)
  - COPD (thin, increased respiratory rate, accessory muscle use)
  - Crohn's disease or ulcerative colitis (abdominal scars, colostomy bag)

> ### BOX 2.73 CAUSES OF CUSHING'S SYNDROME
>
> - Iatrogenic steroid therapy
> - Adrenocortical adenoma
> - Adrenocortical adenocarcinoma
> - ACTH-producing microadenoma (Cushing's disease)
> - ACTH-secreting tumours, e.g. small cell bronchial carcinoma, carcinoid, pancreatic carcinoma (Cushing's disease)

ASSOCIATED DISEASES

- Diabetes mellitus or impaired glucose tolerance
- Hypertension
- Increased risk of heart disease
- Impotence or menstrual disturbance
- Obstructive sleep apnoea
- Carpal tunnel syndrome
- Osteoporosis, vertebral fractures and kyphoscoliosis
- Depression, psychiatric disturbance

INVESTIGATIONS

- 24-hour urinary cortisol
- Low-dose dexamethasone suppression test
- MRI brain may be of use in some cases
- Bilateral inferior petrosal sinus sampling

TREATMENT

- Treat the cause
- To avoid steroid-related osteoporosis give:
  - Calcium and vitamin D
  - Bisphosphonates
  - Hormone replacement therapy or testosterone

ACROMEGALY

Acromegaly is an endocrine disease caused by a growth hormone producing macroadenoma of the pituitary gland. The mass effect of this adenoma may also induce hypopituitarism.

INSPECTION

Hands

- Large, 'doughy'
- 'Spade-like'
- Square-shaped
- Thickened skin
- Carpal tunnel syndrome or scars from release

Face

- 'Coarse' features
- Enlarged ears and nose
- Large tongue
- Increased interdental spacing
- Prognathism
- Prominent supraorbital ridges
- Husky, low pitch voice
- Greasy skin and acne
- Hirsutism

BOX 2.74 COMMON SYMPTOMS OF ACROMEGALY

- Headaches
- Visual field disturbance
- Sweating
- Increased shoe and glove size
- Wedding ring no longer fits
- Dentures become too small
- Features 'coarsen'
- Loss of libido

Eyes

- Bitemporal hemianopia (owing to mass effect at optic chiasm)

Generally

- Goitre
- Gynaecomastia
- Small (or large) testes – depending on degree of hypopituitarism
- Osteoarthritis, kyphosis
- Proximal muscle weakness
- Acanthosis nigricans

ASSOCIATED DISEASES

- Hypopituitarism
- Diabetes mellitus or impaired glucose tolerance
- Hypertension
- Cardiomyopathy
- Increased risk of heart disease
- Colorectal cancer
- Hypercalciuria and renal stones
- Obstructive sleep apnoea
- Carpal tunnel syndrome

BOX 2.75 TREATMENT OF ACROMEGALY

- Somatostatin analogues, e.g. octreotide
- Bromocriptine
- Pegvisomant – growth hormone receptor antagonist
- Radiation if surgery unsuccessful
- Trans-sphenoidal hypophysectomy

INVESTIGATIONS

- Glucose tolerance test – positive test shows lack of suppression and occasionally a paradoxical rise in growth hormone
- Perimetry to delineate visual field defect
- MRI brain
- Anterior pituitary hormone tests to check for hypopituitarism

DIABETES MELLITUS

Diabetes mellitus is a common disease that can be split into two categories:

- Type 1: onset at a younger age (children or young adults), resulting from autoimmune pancreatic β-cell failure, requiring immediate insulin replacement
- Type 2: onset at an older age (many are overweight), resulting from peripheral insulin resistance, requiring a range of treatment from diet control to oral hypoglycaemic agents and insulin

Diabetes may be caused by other diseases such as Cushing's syndrome (see p. 151) or haemochromatosis.

HISTORY

Type 1

- Nausea and vomiting, diarrhoea
- Weight loss
- Polyuria
- Polydipsia
- Dehydration
- Lethargy and fatigue
- Diabetic ketoacidosis

Type 2

- Often asymptomatic
- Lethargy and malaise
- Polyuria
- Polydipsia
- Frequent skin or soft tissue infections
- Symptoms of peripheral neuropathy
- Foot ulcers
- Visual symptoms

INSPECTION

Generally

- Signs of other autoimmune diseases, e.g.:
  - Vitiligo
  - Thyroid disease
  - Rheumatoid arthritis

Eyes

- Diabetic retinopathy and cataract (see p. 90)

Feet

- Ulcers
- Calluses over pressure points
- 'Glove and stocking' peripheral neuropathy
- Charcot's joint (e.g. ankle)

Skin lesions

- Skin ulcers
- Lipodystrophy, e.g. atrophy, hypertrophy at sites of repeated insulin injection – abdomen, thigh
- Necrobiosis lipoidica diabeticorum – well-demarcated oval plaques on shins
- Acanthosis nigricans – velvety, brown/black pigmentation in axillae and groin (many causes including insulin resistance)

BOX 2.76 DIABETIC EMERGENCIES

- Diabetic ketoacidosis – occurs with hyperglycaemia with a lack of insulin in type 1 diabetes – can result in coma or death
- HONK – hyperosmolar non-ketotic coma occurs due to prolonged hyperglycaemia in people with type 2 diabetes – can also be very dangerous
- Hypoglycaemia – can result in seizures, coma or death

INVESTIGATIONS

- Body mass index
- Blood pressure
- Urinalysis: protein, glucose
- U&Es – typically hypokalaemic, hyponatraemia, hyperchloraemic metabolic acidosis (although U&Es may be normal)
- Capillary glucose monitoring (BM)
- Lab blood glucose (fasting)
- Lipid profile (fasting)
- HbA_{1c} (assess blood glucose control)

TREATMENT

Type 1

- Insulin replacement therapy
- Vaccinations
- Education:
  - Frequent BM monitoring – record in a diary
  - Sick days – insulin requirements increase during intercurrent illness
  - Test for urinary ketones when unwell (to rule out diabetic ketoacidosis)
  - Exercise – insulin requirements will be decreased
  - Refrigerate insulin where possible

Type 2

- Education (as above)
- Weight loss, increase physical exercise
- Diet control
- Oral hypoglycaemics ± insulin replacement
- Tight blood pressure control (<140/80 mmHg), e.g. ACE inhibitors
- Monitoring for proteinuria/renal impairment
- Ophthalmology monitoring/referral
- Podiatry

ADDISON'S DISEASE AND HYPOADRENALISM

Hypoadrenalism can occur secondary to a number of causes. Addison's disease refers to hypoadrenalism occurring secondary to adrenal failure leading to deficiency of steroid (cortisol) and mineralocorticoid (aldosterone).

BOX 2.77 CAUSES OF HYPOADRENALISM

- Autoimmune adrenal destruction
- Tuberculosis
- Metastatic adrenal infiltration
- Waterhouse–Friderichsen syndrome (adrenal infarction secondary to septicaemia)
- Adrenal haemorrhage (e.g. anticoagulant therapy)
- Congenital adrenal hyperplasia
- Bilateral adrenalectomy (e.g. metastatic disease)
- HIV
- Fungal infiltration
- Amyloidosis
- Haemochromatosis

HISTORY

- Nausea and vomiting, diarrhoea
- Weight loss
- Lethargy and fatigue
- Sweating
- Headaches
- Hypoglycaemia
- Collapse, loss of conscious, syncope
- Confusion
- Seizures
- Abdominal or leg pain

Note: The latter symptoms may represent a life-threatening Addisonian crisis.

INSPECTION

Generally

- Pigmentation – especially in skin creases (e.g. palms) and scars, nipples and pressure points (e.g. elbows)
- Postural hypotension
- Signs of other autoimmune diseases, e.g.:
  - Vitiligo
  - Thyroid disease
  - Diabetes mellitus
  - Rheumatoid arthritis

Face

- Pigmentation:
  - Buccal mucosa
  - Lips

INVESTIGATIONS

- Urea and electrolytes – typically hyperkalaemic, hyponatraemia, hyperchloraemic metabolic acidosis (although U&Es may be normal)
- Short Synacthen (tetracosactide) test:
  - Synthetic ACTH is administered
  - Plasma is analysed to assess if there is an appropriate rise in cortisol
- Imaging (to elicit cause)
  - Ultrasound scan
  - CT
  - MRI

TREATMENT

- Steroid and mineralocorticoid replacement therapy are the mainstays of management in hypoadrenalism and Addisonian crises.

DERMATOLOGY

SKIN

Examination of the skin is essential as it can provide many clues as to an underlying disease process.

HISTORY

It is important to take a full history when presented with a skin problem. Pay special attention to:

- History of presenting complaint, e.g. when it started, where it is, has it spread, has it changed
- Past medical history, e.g. diabetes, systemic lupus erythematosus, inflammatory bowel disease, atopy

- Drug history, e.g. antibiotics, new detergents
- Social history, e.g. sun exposure, occupation, exposure to animals or plants
- Review of symptoms, e.g. associated swelling, pain, joint problems

EXAMINATION

Introduction

- Gain permission
- Ask about pain
- Expose to underwear
- Position on the couch
- Ensure bright, even lighting

Inspection

- Distribution of rash:
    - Eczema: flexor surfaces, face, hands
    - Psoriasis: extensor surfaces (knees, elbows), scalp, natal cleft
    - Allergic dermatitis: e.g. on hands if exposed to gloves
    - Photosensitive: on areas exposed to the sun, e.g. face, forearms, legs and neck
    - Herpes zoster: distinct dermatomal distribution
    - Bilateral or widespread rash: systemic cause, e.g. viral exanthems
- Morphology of rash:
    - Size
    - Shape – round, oval, target
    - Surface – shiny, crusty
    - Colour – red, salmon pink, silvery, white, yellow, grey
    - Border/edge – well-demarcated, irregular, rolled

Table 2.6 Dermatological terms

Term	Definition
Abscess	A local accumulation of pus
Atrophy	Wasting away/diminution
Bulla	Blister >5 cm
Comedone	Plug of sebaceous and dead skin material stuck in the opening of a hair
Follicle	Open (blackhead) or closed (whitehead)
Erosion	Loss of epithelium
Erythema	Redness of the skin
Hyperpigmentation	Increased pigmentation
Hypopigmentation	Decreased pigmentation
Macule	A small, flat, distinct, coloured area of skin <10 mm in diameter
Nodule	Raised lesion >1 cm (an enlargement of a papule)
Papule	Small, circumscribed, palpable lesion
Plaque	Large elevated solid lesions
Purpura	Non-blanching, haemorrhagic lesions, >3 mm
Pustule	Blister containing pus
Scaling	An increase in the dead cells on the surface of the skin (stratum corneum)
Telangiectasia	Prominent cutaneous dilated blood vessels
Ulcer	Full-thickness loss of epidermis or epithelium, may be covered with a dark coloured crust (eschar)
Vesicle	Small, fluid-filled blister
Wheals	Cutaneous oedema due to leaking capillaries

- Arrangement of rash:
  - Group of papules, e.g. insect bites
  - Clusters, e.g. of vesicles
  - Koebner's phenomenon – predilection for rash in trauma-prone areas

Table 2.7 Cutaneous manifestations of underlying diseases

Signs	Disease
Arthritis/arthropathy/joint deformity	Systemic lupus erythematosus, rheumatoid arthritis, psoriatic arthritis
Tight skin, beak nose, microstomia	Systemic sclerosis
Gottron's papules, heliotrope rash, nailfold telangiectasia	Dermatomyositis
Necrobiosis lipoidica	Diabetes
Erythema nodosum, pyoderma gangrenosum	Inflammatory bowel disease
Acanthosis nigricans	Insulin resistance
Xanthelasma	Hyperlipidaemia
Dermatitis herpetiformis	Coeliac disease
Erythema nodosum	Inflammatory bowel disease
Lupus pernio/erythema nodosum	Sarcoidosis

PSORIASIS

Psoriasis is a common chronic skin disorder affecting up to 2 per cent of the population in the UK. It occurs most frequently between adolescence and middle age, as a result of increased skin cell synthesis, though the underlying cause for this is not known.

BOX 2.78 TYPES OF PSORIASIS

- Plaque: the most common form comprising scaly plaques over extensor surfaces including elbows and knees. This type can also affect the scalp, nails, natal cleft and umbilicus
- Guttate: (from the Latin *gutta*, a drop) occurs in children and teenagers often after a streptococcal infection. Plaques are widespread and tear-drop shaped – they often resolve fully
- Pustular: pustules occur in place of plaques and can affect various areas of the body, e.g. palmar-plantar pustular psoriasis
- Erythrodermic: this severe form of the disease can be potentially life-threatening causing a widespread erythematous rash

---

EXAMINATION

- Plaques are:
  - Circular
  - Well defined
  - Erythematous/salmon-coloured
  - Silvery
  - Scaly
  - Classically located over extensor surfaces, i.e. elbows and knees, but also scalp and natal cleft, chest and trunk
- Koebner's phenomenon: propensity for plaques to occur over areas of trauma

Other manifestations include:

- Nail pitting and onycholysis
- Coexisting arthropathy (see p. 126; rheumatoid arthritis/psoriatic arthritis), e.g.:
  - Symmetrical inflammatory small joint involvement
  - Large joint arthropathy
  - Arthritis mutilans (with telescoping of digits)

BOX 2.79 SKIN DISEASES EXHIBITING KOEBNER'S PHENOMENON

- Psoriasis
- Lichen planus
- Vitiligo

- Molluscum contagiosum
- Bullous pemphigoid

INVESTIGATIONS

- Diagnosis is usually clinically based on appearance and distribution of plaques
- Biopsy rarely needed but can be helpful if the presentation is not typical

TREATMENT

- Topical agents:
  - Emollients
  - Salicylic acid
  - Coal tar
  - Vitamin D analogues, e.g. calcipotriol
  - Dithranol
  - Steroids
- Oral therapies:
  - Methotrexate
  - Ciclosporin
- UVB phototherapy

ECZEMA

This is a common skin disorder, also referred to as dermatitis. Its prevalence is around 1 per cent of adults and 20 per cent of children in the UK.

HISTORY

Patient with eczema may also have a history of:

- Asthma
- Hayfever
- Familial tendency
- Known sensitivities, e.g. house dust-mites, pollen, foods or pets

EXAMINATION

Skin lesions that are classically:

- Dry
- Scaly
- Itchy
- Lichenified
- Erythematous

If secondary infection has occurred swelling and exudate may be noted.

Distribution of rash:

- Although it can be widespread the classical pattern is that affecting flexor surfaces, e.g. wrists, elbows, knees
- In young children it may also affect the face, neck and nappy area

---

BOX 2.80 DIAGNOSIS OF ECZEMA

- >12 months itchy skin lesions
- History (or family history) of asthma or hayfever
- Erythematous, scaly rash
- Flexor distribution (children may involve forehead, cheeks, arms and legs)

INVESTIGATIONS

- Diagnosis is usually clinical and based on appearance and distribution of rash
- Biopsy – occasionally required if diagnosis is not clear

TREATMENT

- Avoid precipitating factors, e.g. detergents
- Topical emollients
- Topical steroids
- Antihistamines
- PUVA therapy
- Immunosuppressive agents for severe cases, e.g. methotrexate, tacrolimus
- Antibiotics for concurrent skin infection

MALIGNANT SKIN LESIONS

These can be broadly divided into melanomas and non-melanomatous skin cancers, e.g. BCC and SCC:

- Melanomas account for approximately 10 per cent of skin cancers in the UK
- Basal cell carcinoma (BCC) is the most common at roughly 70 per cent
- Squamous cell carcinoma (SCC) accounts for around 20 per cent

HISTORY

- New or changing papule/macule (e.g. mole), on sun-exposed areas, with or without:
  - Itching
  - Ulceration
  - Discharge/bleeding

    ○   Altered pigmentation
    ○   Increasing size
    ○   Scaling
- Drug history (see Box 2.81)
- Social history including occupation (see Box 2.81)

BOX 2.81 RISK FACTORS FOR DEVELOPING MALIGNANT SKIN LESIONS

- Sun (UV) exposure: occupational, e.g. sailors, recreational, e.g. suntanning
- Sunbed use
- Fair hair, fair skin, blue eyes
- Numerous moles (e.g. >20) and freckles
- Previous severe sunburn ± blistering
- Radiotherapy burns
- Family history
- Drug history, e.g. doxycycline causes increased light sensitivity
- Industrial toxin exposure
- Immunosuppression, e.g. HIV, immunosuppressant therapy

EXAMINATION

Basal cell carcinoma

- Skin lesion, most frequently on the face, exhibiting:
  - Flesh-coloured papule
  - 'Pearly' appearance with telangiectasia
  - Raised border
  - Central ulceration
  - Rarely: waxy yellow/white papule

Squamous cell carcinoma

- New papule/macule, on sun-exposed area, with or without:
  - Itching
  - Ulceration
  - Discharge/bleeding
  - Altered pigmentation
  - Increasing size
  - Scaling/crusting
- Cluster of vesicular-like lesions
- Skin lesion, most frequently on the face or other sun-exposed areas (may also occur in perianal regions, penis or inside mouth)

Melanoma

- New mole
- Change in appearance of existing mole, using 'ABCDE' criteria
  - A: asymmetry
  - B: border – irregular
  - C: colours – two or more

- ○ D: diameter >6 mm
- ○ E: elevation above the surface of the skin
- Other signs:
  - ○ Lymphadenopathy (local/distant)
  - ○ Evidence of distant metastases, e.g. lung, liver

INVESTIGATIONS

- Excision biopsy
- Lymph node biopsy
- CT scan if evidence/suspicion of metastases

TREATMENT

- Prevention:
  - ○ Avoid sun exposure, especially in the middle of the day
  - ○ Sunblock
- Removal:
  - ○ Multidisciplinary team approach (e.g. surgeon, dermatologist, pathologist, oncologist)
  - ○ Topical immunotherapy
  - ○ Cryotherapy
  - ○ Surgical excision
  - ○ Radio/chemotherapy

PROGNOSIS

- BCC
  - ○ The prognosis is generally good with an over 90 per cent cure rate
- SCC
  - ○ This carries a slightly poorer prognosis, with around 5 per cent metastasizing
- Melanoma
  - ○ Prognosis depends on stage of lesion at presentation. It carries the greatest risk of mortality of all the skin cancers. The earliest lesions are usually curable but those that have spread deeper into the skin often carry a grim prognosis

NEUROFIBROMATOSIS

This autosomal dominant disease is a neurocutaneous condition. It can affect almost every organ of the body and there is a wide range of severity. There are two main types:

- Neurofibromatosis type 1 – von Recklinghausen's disease (chromosome 17)
- Neurofibromatosis type 2 – central neurofibromatosis (chromosome 22)

INSPECTION

- Multiple soft (or firm) neurofibromas
  - ○ Subcutaneous
  - ○ Mobile
  - ○ Along peripheral nerves

- ○ May be a fusiform enlargement, i.e. plexiform neurofibromas (specifically in neurofibromatosis type 1)
- Multiple 'café au lait spots' – brown macules
  - ○ Must have six or more
  - ○ Measure >5 mm in diameter in children or >15 mm in post-pubertal patients
- Axillary freckling
- Lisch nodules in the iris:
  - ○ Melanocytic hamartomas
  - ○ Dome-shaped
  - ○ Seen best with a slit lamp
  - ○ Present in all patients over 20 years
- Neurological abnormalities:
  - ○ Acoustic neuromas (vestibular schwannomas) and subsequent deafness (especially in neurofibromatosis type 2)
  - ○ Meningiomas, astrocytomas, etc.
  - ○ Spinal cord compression (from either skeletal abnormality or neurofibroma)
  - ○ Optic nerve gliomas
  - ○ Learning difficulties, below average IQ
  - ○ Epilepsy
- Renal artery stenosis
- Phaeochromocytomas
- Bone involvement – multiple possible defects, e.g. bowing of tibia
- Scars from operations for any of the above, e.g. excision of nodule

---

BOX 2.82 DIAGNOSTIC CRITERIA FOR NEUROFIBROMATOSIS TYPE 1 AND 2

Neurofibromatosis type 1 (two or more features):
- Two or more neurofibromas (or one plexiform)
- Six or more café au lait macules
- Axillary (or groin) freckling
- Two or more Lisch nodules
- Bony lesion
- First degree relative with the above

Neurofibromatosis type 2 (these patients often have fewer skin manifestations):
- Bilateral acoustic neuromas
- First degree relative with neurofibromatosis type 2
- Either a unilateral acoustic neuroma or two of:
  - ○ neurofibroma
  - ○ meningioma
  - ○ schwannoma

Source: Acoustic Neuroma. National Institutes of Health Consensus Development Conference Statement, 11–13 December 1991

FURTHER INVESTIGATIONS

- Screen relatives regularly for hearing problems (especially in neurofibromatosis type 2)
- Blood pressure (phaeochromocytoma, renal artery stenosis)
- Wood's lamp may aid identification of macules on pale skin

MARFAN'S DISEASE

This autosomal dominant disease is caused by a mutation in the fibrillin gene on chromosome 15 resulting in a connective tissue disorder.

INSPECTION

Musculoskeletal system

- Tall stature: arm span greater than height (or pubis to sole distance > pubis to vertex)
- Kyphoscoliosis
- Pectus excavatum
- Reduced musculature
- Reduced elbow extension
- Arachnodactyly: long, spider-like fingers and toes

BOX 2.83 DIAGNOSING ARACHNODACTYLY

- Steinberg's thumb sign: when the thumb is fully opposed against the palm, in a closed fist, it stretches beyond the ulnar border of the hand
- Walker's wrist sign: overlap of the thumb and little finger when placed around the opposite wrist

---

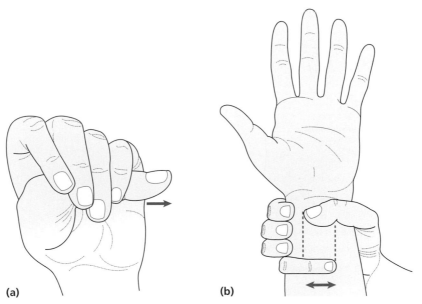

(a)   (b)

Figure 2.24 (a) Steinberg's thumb sign; (b) Walker's wrist sign

Eyes

- Blue sclera
- Upwards lens subluxation (seen with slit lamp)
- Cataract
- Retinal detachment

Cardiovascular

- Mitral valve prolapse
- Aortic root dilation
- Aortic dissection
- Aortic regurgitation
- Aortic aneurysms

Other

- High-arched palate
- Hernias

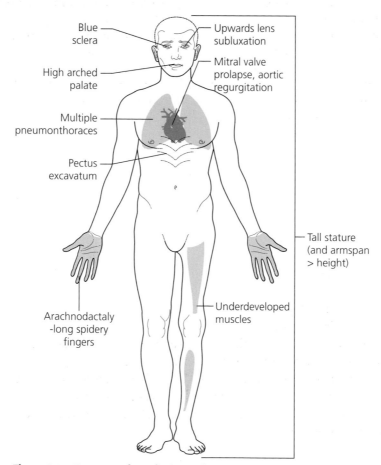

Figure 2.25 Features of Marfan's syndrome

INVESTIGATIONS

Marfan's is essentially a clinical diagnosis. Useful investigations include:

- Gene analysis
- Chest X-ray
- Echocardiogram
- CT/MRI aorta

Procedures

OBSERVATIONS

INDICATIONS

- Observations include:
  - Temperature
  - Blood pressure
  - Pulse rate
  - Oxygen saturation
  - Respiratory rate
- They must be assessed in all new hospital admissions and at regular intervals during an inpatient stay depending on the severity of the condition
- Observations are vital in the assessment of the acutely deteriorating patient
- Hourly urine output is sometimes included as part of regular observations, particularly in patients with cardiac or renal failure or in patients in shock and in higher care environments

CONTRAINDICATIONS

- Patient refusal despite careful explanation of risks and benefits

PREPARATION

- Explain procedure
- Obtain consent
- Assemble:
  - Calibrated sphygmomanometer, stethoscope and alcohol wipe
  - Watch with seconds displayed

   ○   Pulse oximeter
   ○   Temperature probe – disposable oral sticks (TempaDOTs) or tympanic ear probes are commonly used

POSITIONING

Assessments can be performed with a patient lying, sitting or standing.

TECHNIQUE

- Identify the patient and obtain consent
- Wash hands

Heart rate

- Pulse rate should be measured manually by palpation of the radial, brachial or carotid pulse
- Inaccuracies may occur in patients with atrial fibrillation, and an apical heart rate should be measured in these patients
- Automated observation machines will provide the user with a heart rate, taken from the saturation trace (again inaccuracies occur with atrial fibrillation)

Blood pressure

- See page 169
- This can be performed with a sphygmomanometer or an automated device

Temperature

- Can be measured orally under the tongue, using disposable sticks
- Can be measured with ear probe devices that measure the temperature at the tympanic membrane
- Other more invasive techniques include rectal and oesophageal temperatures
- Axillary temperatures are rarely used due to inaccuracies in their readings (up to 1° below core temperature)

Oxygen saturations

- Oxygen saturations are measured with a pulse oximeter
- A pulse oximeter measures the transmission of light through a pulsatile vascular bed and is calibrated to give a saturation reading and thus a measurement of oxygenation
- The probe is placed over the fingertip ideally on the opposite hand to the blood pressure cuff which will disrupt readings when inflated
- Coloured nail varnish must be removed as this can also cause inaccuracies
- The probe should be left in place for at least 30 seconds to obtain a stable trace
- If the peripheries are poorly perfused, measurements can be taken with probes adapted for the ear lobe

Respiratory rate

- Respiratory rate should be measured for at least 30 seconds to gain an accurate count
- It can be performed while the other observations are being obtained and the distraction of the patient with these procedures will provide a more accurate result

- Follow-up:
  - Wash your hands before moving on
  - All observations should be documented with a date and time
  - If any abnormalities are found the reading should be repeated and a senior informed
  - The assessor should be aware of changes in the trend of readings as much as the actual values themselves

NORMAL ADULT RANGES

- Heart rate 60–100 beats/minute
- Blood pressure 90–140 mmHg systolic/60–90 mmHg diastolic
- Temperature 36–37.5 °C
- Oxygen saturations >95 per cent
- Respiratory rate 10–16 breaths/minute

BLOOD PRESSURE

INDICATIONS

All patients should have a blood pressure measurement recorded on admission, and as part of regular inpatient observations at a frequency dictated by the severity of their illness.

CONTRAINDICATIONS

- Patient refusal despite careful explanation of risks and benefits

PREPARATION

- Explain procedure
- Obtain consent
- Assemble:
  - Calibrated sphygmomanometer
  - Blood pressure cuff – select a size appropriate for the patient: the bladder should encircle 80 per cent of the arm
  - Stethoscope
  - Alcohol wipe

POSITIONING

- Ideally the patient should be sitting for 10 minutes prior to assessment
- The arm should be extended at the level of the heart and supported in a relaxed position, e.g. on a table or a pillow
- All outer clothing should be removed from the upper arm

LANDMARKS

- Palpate the brachial artery, which can be felt in the medial aspect of the antecubital fossa

TECHNIQUE

- Identify the patient and obtain informed consent
- Wash hands
- Place the cuff around the upper arm ensuring all the air is released from the cuff
- The artery arrow, which lies in the centre of the cuff bladder, should be aligned with the brachial artery
- Inflate the cuff while palpating the radial pulse
- The moment when the radial pulse can no longer be felt is the estimated systolic pressure
- Deflate the cuff
- Clean the diaphragm of the stethoscope with the alcohol wipe
- Inflate the cuff to 20 mmHg above the previously estimated systolic pressure while palpating the radial pulse
- Place the diaphragm over the brachial artery and slowly release the cuff pressure by 2 mmHg every second
- The first tapping sound that will be heard is known as Korotkoff phase 1 (see Box 3.1) and represents the systolic pressure
- The pressure should continue to be released and the moment that all the sounds disappear in their entirety, known as Korotkoff phase 5, represents the diastolic pressure
- Remove the cuff
- Wash hands
- Follow-up:
  - Document:
    - The systolic and diastolic pressures
    - The arm from which they were taken
    - The patient's position at the time of measurement
  - If postural pressures are required, measure the supine pressure before the standing pressure
  - Occasionally pressure measurements will be required from both arms for a comparison when assessing, for example, for thoracic aortic dissection

---

BOX 3.1 KOROTKOFF PHASES

- First phase – the first audible tapping sounds begin (corresponds with the systolic pressure)
- Second phase – a soft pulsation is heard
- Third phase – a crisper beat is heard
- Fourth phase – the beats change into a blowing sound
- Fifth phase – the beats become inaudible and correspond to the diastolic pressure

---

COMPLICATIONS

- Inaccurate readings from:
  - A poorly calibrated sphygmomanometer
  - Incorrect cuff size
  - Atrial fibrillation
  - Patients with hyperdynamic circulations, e.g. during pregnancy, can be difficult to assess

- Failure to palpate the radial pulse can lead to the missing of a 'silent gap' in patients with very high blood pressures, and, as a result, inaccurately low pressures are recorded for these patients

BLOOD (CAPILLARY) GLUCOSE MEASUREMENT

INDICATIONS

- Regular assessment in any diabetic patient
- Assessment of any newly admitted patient
- Assessment of any acutely deteriorating patient

CONTRAINDICATIONS

- Patient refusal despite careful explanation of risks and benefits
- Localized infection (change site)

PREPARATION

- Explain procedure
- Obtain consent
- Assemble:
  - Disposable tray
  - Alcohol gel for cleaning hands
  - Gloves
  - Alcohol swab
  - Calibrated glucometer and testing sticks
  - Lancet
  - Sharps bin
  - Appropriate dressing, e.g. cotton wool ball

POSITIONING

- Sit patient comfortably
- Extend the arm on a pillow, below the level of the heart

LANDMARKS

- Side of any fingertip (try to avoid the pulp)

TECHNIQUE

- Turn on the glucometer and insert an in-date testing stick
- Wash hands and don gloves
- Clean area and allow to dry
- Squeeze the fingertip between the thumb and index finger
- Pierce the skin with a lancet (these vary and are usually spring loaded)
- Place the lancet in a sharps bin immediately after use
- Continue to squeeze the finger until a droplet of blood is seen
- Place the testing stick next to the droplet of blood which will be drawn into the stick
- The glucometer will 'beep' when sufficient blood has been collected

- Apply pressure over the puncture site with a dressing until the bleeding stops
- Dispose of the testing stick and switch off the glucometer when the result is obtained
- Wash hands
- Follow-up – document the time of sampling and the result in the notes

Note: This is a capillary blood sample. Fasting glucose samples for formal assessment of diabetes require a venous sample obtained by venesection.

COMPLICATIONS

- Failure to obtain a reading, e.g. defective glucometer, not enough blood for sample
- Inaccurate results owing to contamination of fingers

VENEPUNCTURE

INDICATIONS

- Venous blood sampling
- Therapeutic venesection, e.g. haemochromatosis

CONTRAINDICATIONS

- Patient refusal despite careful explanation of risks and benefits
- Localized infection (change site)

PREPARATION

- Explain procedure
- Obtain consent
- Assemble:
  - Disposable tray
  - Alcohol gel for cleaning hands
  - Disposable tourniquet
  - Gloves
  - Alcohol swab
  - Needle and vacutainer (connect together before use)
  - Appropriate blood bottles
  - Sharps bin
  - Dressing and tape to secure
  - Blood test request form

POSITIONING

- Sit patient comfortably
- Support the extended arm on a pillow

LANDMARKS

- Identify a suitable vein, usually in the antecubital fossa
- This is most commonly the median cubital vein; the basilic and cephalic vein can be used as alternatives
- Avoid sampling from a functioning arteriovenous fistula

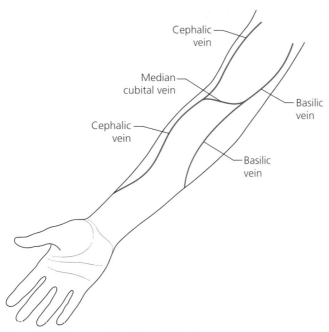

Figure 3.1 Venepuncture sites of the forearm

TECHNIQUE

- Wash hands and don gloves
- Apply a tourniquet approximately 5 cm above the intended puncture site, tight enough to occlude venous return, but not arterial flow into the arm
- Clean the area with an alcohol wipe and allow to dry
- Insert the needle – bevel up – along the line of the identified vein at a 15° angle while tethering the skin with your free hand
- Advance into the vein – you may feel a 'pop' when you enter it
- Fill each bottle individually, citrate (blue clotting) first, if required
- Invert each blood bottle gently to mix blood with bottle medium
- Release tourniquet
- Remove the needle and place directly into a sharps bin
- Apply pressure over the puncture site with a dressing for 1 minute
- Secure the dressing with tape
- Wash hands
- Follow-up:
  - Label blood bottles at the bedside confirming patient details
  - Send to the lab
  - Ensure results are checked

COMPLICATIONS

- Failure/difficulty locating vein
- Infection (rare)
- Bleeding
- Haematoma

BLOOD CULTURES

Blood cultures are taken in a similar fashion to venepuncture.

- They are performed when bacteraemia is suspected: patients are usually septic. Blood cultures are especially important in the diagnosis of endocarditis
- When sampling for infective endocarditis, three sets of cultures need to be taken from three different sites at different times ideally coinciding with the times of peak fever
- The equipment and technique are identical to venepuncture with the exception that you will require one anaerobic and one aerobic culture bottle
- Clean the tops of the collection bottles with separate alcohol swabs and allow to dry
- A non-touch technique is essential (the site of puncture should not be touched after cleaning)
- Perform venepuncture. Do not change the needle on the syringe
- Inoculate the blood into the anaerobic bottle first and then the aerobic bottle. Aim for 10 mL of blood in each bottle
- Arrange for porter to take the samples to the laboratory urgently for incubation
- Ensure results are checked; they may take 24–72 hours

PERIPHERAL VENOUS CANNULATION

INDICATIONS

- Administration of:
  - Intravenous fluids
  - Drugs
  - Blood and blood products

CONTRAINDICATIONS

- Patient refusal despite careful explanation of risks and benefits
- Localized infection (change site)

PREPARATION

- Explain procedure
- Obtain consent
- Assemble:
  - Disposable tray
  - Alcohol gel for cleaning hands
  - Disposable tourniquet
  - Gloves
  - Chlorhexidine swab
  - Venous cannula: select appropriate size according to indication
  - 10 mL syringe
  - 10 mL 0.9 per cent saline
  - Sharps bin
  - Cannula dressing

POSITIONING

- Sit patient comfortably
- Support the extended arm on a pillow

LANDMARKS

- Identify a suitable vein, classically the cephalic ('houseman's') vein on the lateral aspect of the forearm. Alternatives include the dorsum of the hand and antecubital fossa
- Ideally insert into the non-dominant arm
- Try to avoid insertion near joints that can obstruct intravenous fluid flow when flexed
- Avoid insertion into an arteriovenous fistula

TECHNIQUE

- Wash hands and don gloves
- Draw up 10 mL saline into the syringe
- Apply the tourniquet approximately 5 cm above the intended puncture site, tight enough to occlude venous return but not arterial flow into the arm
- Clean the area and allow to dry
- Insert the cannula along the line of the identified vein at a 15° angle while tethering the skin with the free hand
- You may feel a 'pop' when you enter the vein and you will see blood 'flash back' up the cannula
- Advance another 2 mm
- Withdraw the needle, while holding the cannula still, ensuring blood is filling the cannula sheath
- Advance cannula sheath smoothly into the vein
- Release tourniquet
- Remove the needle and place directly into a sharps bin. Compress the vein at the tip of the cannula while doing this (prevents unnecessary blood spillage)
- Apply bung
- Secure with a cannula dressing
- Flush cannula with saline, this syringe should depress easily and the patient may feel a cold sensation up the arm. If painful, cannula is not within vein and must be removed
- Wash hands
- Follow-up:
    - Label the cannula with the date inserted
    - Document in the notes the size of cannula, site and date of insertion

COMPLICATIONS

- Failure, difficulty locating vein
- Extravasation of drugs or fluids – 'tissuing' of the cannula: fluid flowing into the subcutaneous tissue
- Bleeding/haematoma
- Infection
- Nerve injury
- Accidental arterial puncture

ARTERIAL BLOOD GAS SAMPLING

INDICATIONS

- Rapid assessment of the acutely ill patient
- Assessment of:
  - Oxygenation/ventilation
  - Acid–base status
  - Electrolytes
  - Haemoglobin concentration (when rapid result needed)

CONTRAINDICATIONS

- Patient refusal despite careful explanation of risks and benefits
- Localized infection (change site)
- Failed Allen's test (see Box 3.2) if sampling from the radial artery

---

BOX 3.2 ALLEN'S TEST

- Ask the patient to make a fist and then raise the hand for 30 seconds
- Occlude ulnar and radial arteries with your thumbs
- When the fist is released the hand should appear blanched
- Release pressure over the ulnar artery and colour should return to the hand within 7 seconds if the ulnar collateral supply is sufficient, i.e. it is deemed safe to sample from and potentially disrupt the radial artery supply

---

PREPARATION

- Explain procedure
- Obtain consent
- Assemble:
  - Disposable tray
  - Alcohol gel for cleaning hands
  - Disposable tourniquet
  - Gloves
  - Alcohol swab
  - Lidocaine 1 per cent (in a syringe with an orange needle)
  - Heparinized arterial blood sampling syringe and needle
  - Sharps bin
  - Dressing and tape to secure

POSITIONING

- Sit the patient comfortably
- Extend the wrist on a pillow
- Place a protective sheet, e.g. incontinence pad, under the wrist

LANDMARKS

- Palpate the radial pulse

- Assess collateral circulation by performing Allen's test (see Box 3.2)
- An alternative site is the femoral artery
- The brachial artery is not recommended since it is an end artery

TECHNIQUE

- Wash hands and don gloves
- Draw up lidocaine into a syringe
- Clean the area and allow to dry
- Introduce a bleb of lidocaine subcutaneously over the intended puncture site
- Allow it to have its effect for 2 minutes
- Palpate the artery with index and middle finger
- **Note:** be aware of different sampling syringes some of which require priming prior to insertion
- Insert the needle at a 45° angle, bevel up, immediately next to the tip of the index finger along the line of the pulse
- Advance until blood begins to fill the syringe
- Remove the needle when the syringe is filled with at least 1 mL of blood
- Apply pressure with a dressing over the puncture site for at least 2 minutes
- Remove the needle from the syringe and cover with a cap
- Expel excess air from the syringe through the cap
- Place the needle directly into a sharps bin
- Secure the dressing with tape
- Wash hands
- Follow-up:
  - Analyze the sample immediately
  - If there is any delay in analyzing the sample place the syringe in ice
  - Document the procedure and results in the notes
  - Ensure you document the amount of oxygen inspired (FiO_2)

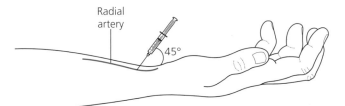

Figure 3.2 Angle of insertion of needle for arterial blood gas sampling

COMPLICATIONS

- Failure, difficulty locating artery
- Bleeding/haematoma
- Infection
- Nerve damage
- Ischaemia of tissues supplied by artery
- Thromboembolic events

MID-STREAM URINE (MSU) SAMPLING

INDICATIONS

- Suspected urinary infection
- Assessment of sepsis of unknown origin
- Assessment of any acutely unwell patient
- Assessment for haematuria/proteinuria
- Screening for myoglobinuria

CONTRAINDICATIONS

- Patient refusal despite careful explanation of risks and benefits

PREPARATION

- Explain procedure
- Obtain consent
- Assemble:
  - Disposable tray
  - Gloves
  - Urinalysis stick and container

TECHNIQUE

- Ask the patient for a freshly voided sample in a clean sample pot
- Wash your hands
- Don gloves
- Identify the type of sample (see below) and patient details
- Dip the urinalysis stick into the sample, ensuring each reagent block is immersed for 1–2 seconds
- Hold the stick horizontally and tap off excess urine
- Wait for the appropriate time to interpret each block according to the container (ranges from 30 seconds to 2 minutes)
- Compare the colour of each square of reagent to the colour chart on the bottle
- Note down the result for each reagent block
- **Note**: some hospitals have an electronic urinalysis machine into which the stick is inserted and the result is printed
- Dispose of the testing stick and sample appropriately
- Wash hands
- Follow-up:
  - Document the result in the patient's notes, including the type of sample obtained
  - Send the sample for microscopy, sensitivity and culture if appropriate

COMPLICATIONS

- False-positive/-negative results (see p. 221)

> **BOX 3.3 TYPES OF URINE SAMPLE**
>
> - Mid-stream
> - Catheter urine
> - Bag urine (mainly paediatrics)
> - Suprapubic catheter urine
> - Early morning

URETHRAL CATHETERIZATION

INDICATIONS

- Urinary retention
- Neuro-axial blockade, e.g. spinal anaesthesia
- Urological surgical intervention, e.g. three-way irrigation catheter for bladder washout
- Delivery of medications, e.g. chemotherapy
- Accurate urine output measurement

CONTRAINDICATIONS

- Patient refusal despite careful explanation of risks and benefits
- Urethral injury, trauma or anatomical abnormality
- Penile anatomical abnormality

PREPARATION

- Explain procedure
- Obtain consent
- Assemble:
  - Two pairs of gloves
  - Sterile drape
  - Gauze swabs
  - Sterile saline for cleaning
  - Galley pot
  - Kidney dish
  - Lidocaine jelly
  - Sterile water for balloon inflation
  - Appropriate catheter and urine collection bag

POSITIONING

- Semi-recumbent position
- Clothes from waist down removed

LANDMARKS

- Male: retract foreskin, locate meatus
- Female: part labia, locate superior-most orifice

TECHNIQUE
Male

- Obtain consent and explain procedure

- Open pack onto trolley and catheter onto pack (keeping its internal packaging on)
- Note the volume of sterile water required to inflate balloon on insertion
- With both pairs of sterile gloves on, hold the penis with gauze in your left hand and after retracting the foreskin, clean the meatus with saline soaked gauze
- Place the sterile drape over the patient, passing the penis through a hole in the centre, to keep sterile
- While holding the penis upwards inject as much local anaesthetic jelly as possible, and hold syringe in meatus for 3 minutes to prevent gel from leaking back
- Dispose of outer gloves
- Open tip of catheter covering and without touching it, insert slowly, peeling back the plastic as you proceed
- Insert catheter as far as the bifurcation and position opening over kidney bowel, between the patient's legs
- Observe for urine flow, indicating tip of catheter is in bladder
- Inject the 10 mL of sterile water into the balloon, watching the patient's face for discomfort
- Pull back the catheter gently until it meets the resistance of the balloon and connect collection bag
- Replace the foreskin
- Document the procedure in the patient's notes, specifying the type, serial number, residual urine volume drained and volume of water injected

Female

Female catheterization is very similar to male. The preparation though is slightly different:

- Take consent and prepare the trolley as above – a shorter catheter is often used due to the shorter length of the female urethra
- Part the labia and clean with the saline swab from top to bottom
- Inject approximately 5 mL of local anaesthetic jelly into the urethra and continue as above

COMPLICATIONS

- Failure to pass catheter, e.g. prostatic enlargement
- Haematuria: urethral injury/trauma
- Stricture formation
- Urinary tract infection
- False passage

NASOGASTRIC TUBE INSERTION

Both nursing staff and doctors can carry out this simple procedure.

INDICATIONS

- Bowel obstruction
- Gastric outlet obstruction
- Enteral feeding and drug administration (fine bore tube)

CONTRAINDICATIONS

- Patient refusal despite careful explanation of risks and benefits
- Base of skull fractures
- Facial fractures
- Unstable cervical spine injury
- Gastric bypass surgery
- Oesophageal varices
- Coagulopathy
- Laryngectomy
- Compromised airway

PREPARATION

- Obtain consent
- Explain procedure to patient
- Appropriate size tube (preferably refrigerated to keep stiff)
  - Large bore for drainage in bowel obstruction (Ryle's tube)
  - Fine bore for feeding
- Lubricating jelly
- Glass of water
- Bladder syringe
- Tape to secure
- Drainage bag

POSITIONING

- Sit the patient upright
- Stand next to the patient

LANDMARKS

- Check the nostrils for patency
- The right nostril is believed to be larger and therefore more appropriate

TECHNIQUE

- Pass the lubricated tube into the nostril, horizontally, until it hits the posterior pharyngeal wall
- Continue to advance the tube, asking the patient to take sips of water and swallow the tube down
- Pass the tube until it reaches roughly 40 cm at the nose and secure
- Aspirate from the tube using the bladder syringe to confirm placement, using pH paper to assess pH <4 (only useful if patient is *not* taking proton pump inhibitors or antacids)
- If the nasogastric tube is for drainage, attach a bag, ensuring the tap is closed
- If the pH results are inconclusive, order a chest X-ray to confirm correct position below the diaphragm, in the stomach

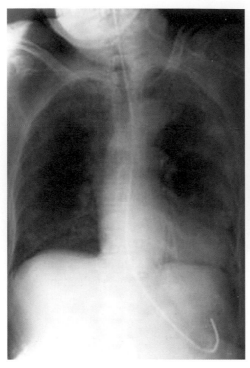

(a)

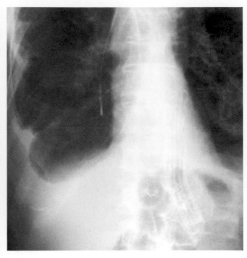

(b)

Figure 3.3 Chest X-ray showing (a) correct and (b) misplaced nasogastric tube in the right bronchus

COMPLICATIONS

- Failure
- Epistaxis, pharyngeal wall injury
- Tracheal placement
- Oesophageal or gastric rupture
- Oesophagitis
- Stricture formation
- Pharyngeal necrosis

JOINT ASPIRATION (ARTHROCENTESIS)

Examination of joint effusion fluid is essential in isolating the diagnosis and therefore the appropriate treatment pathway.

INDICATIONS

- Diagnosis:
  - Septic arthritis (cloudy fluid)
  - Haemarthrosis (blood-stained fluid)
  - Gout or pseudogout (cloudy fluid)
  - Inflammatory arthritis (cloudy fluid)
- Therapeutic:
  - Intra-articular steroid injection
  - Drainage of haemarthrosis or septic joint

CONTRAINDICATIONS

- Patient refusal despite careful explanation of risks and benefits
- Infection near the site
- Coagulopathy, anticoagulation
- Joint prosthesis

PREPARATION

- Explain procedure
- Obtain consent
- Assemble:
  - Sterile pack and gloves
  - Chlorhexidine cleaning solution
  - Appropriate needles and syringe
  - 1 per cent or 2 per cent lidocaine
  - Sterile specimen pots
  - Grey fluoride oxalate glucose vacuum sample bottle

POSITIONING

- Position patient on a bed with the joint, e.g. knee, well supported

LANDMARKS

- For the knee use a lateral approach
- Mark a point 1 cm above and lateral to the superolateral aspect of the patella

TECHNIQUE

- Clean with chlorhexidine solution from centre outwards
- Infiltrate with lidocaine and orange needle, subcutaneously
- Advance the needle, changing it to a green one, aspirating and injecting as you go until joint fluid is aspirated
- After allowing the local anaesthetic to have its effect, enter the same route with a 20 mL syringe and green needle without touching the site
- Aspirate as you advance until joint fluid flows back easily
- Collect as much as required for analysis or until dryness for symptomatic relief
- Cover wound with a small dressing
- Record the procedure, amount of lidocaine used, amount of fluid aspirated and its colour and consistency
- Send samples to laboratory (see Box 3.4)

BOX 3.4 JOINT ASPIRATION INVESTIGATIONS

Microscopy and culture organisms
- Cell count – red blood cells, white blood cells, pus cells
- Crystals – gout (negatively birefringent, needle-shaped) pseudogout (positively birefringent, rhomboid shaped)

COMPLICATIONS

- Unsuccessful tap
- Pain
- Infection
- Bleeding, haematoma

LUMBAR PUNCTURE

INDICATIONS

- Cerebrospinal fluid (CSF) sampling, e.g. for suspected meningitis
- Diagnosis of subarachnoid haemorrhage
- Injection of intrathecal drugs, e.g. chemotherapy agents
- Therapeutic tap to reduce intracranial pressure

CONTRAINDICATIONS

Absolute:

- Patient refusal despite careful explanation of risks and benefits
- Evidence of raised intracranial pressure (ICP) – lumbar puncture could cause coning
- Bleeding diathesis/full anticoagulant therapy (risk of bleeding, haematoma)

Relative:

- Evidence of abnormal anatomy (risk of injuring spine/nerves)
- Local source of infection

PREPARATION

Note: A computed tomography (CT) scan of the brain may be indicated pre-procedure to rule out raised ICP

- Explain procedure
- Obtain consent
- Assemble:
  - Chlorhexidine or iodine solution
  - Sterile pack and gloves
  - Blunt spinal needle
  - Local anaesthetic, e.g. 2 per cent lidocaine
  - Needles (orange and green) and syringe
  - Four sterile collection pots (to be immediately labelled 1–4 afterwards, in order of sampling)
  - Two grey top glucose-measuring blood bottles
  - A small dressing
  - A manometer

POSITIONING

- Lie the patient in the left lateral position
- Ask them to curl up tightly, in the fetal position
- Encourage them to lie still even when they feel the initial injection

LANDMARKS

- Locate Tuffier's line (an imaginary line between the iliac crests)
  - This corresponds with roughly L3/4 (the spinal cord ends at L1/2)
- Feel the space between the spinous processes, in the centre of the back

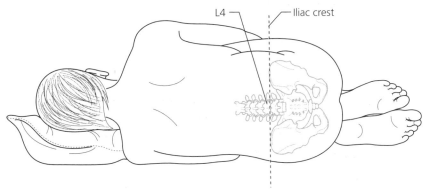

Figure 3.4 Tuffier's line

TECHNIQUE

- Infiltrate subcutaneously, and then more deeply with 5–10 mL of lidocaine
- Allow it to have its effect for 3–5 minutes
- Insert the spinal needle between the spinous processes, in the midline, heading slightly cephalad towards the umbilicus
  - You pass through skin, subcutaneous tissue, supraspinous ligament, and interspinous ligament, and will feel the 'cheese-like' resistance of the ligamentum flavum
  - A 'pop' may be felt when the dura is breeched and the needle is in the intrathecal space
  - CSF should drip freely from the needle on removing the introducer
  - Attach the manometer (you may need a second pair of hands to help with this)
  - Record the highest value at which it settles (normal ~6–20 cmH$_2$O)
  - Take four samples and one in the glucose bottle, roughly five drops in each
  - Ensure you take a serum glucose sample at the same time
- Follow-up:
  - Recommend the patient lies flat for roughly 1 hour post procedure
  - Explain post-lumbar puncture headache, treat as needed with analgesia
  - Send samples 1 and 3 for microscopy cell count and culture
  - Send sample 2 to biochemistry for protein measurement and xanthochromia, if indicated
  - Send the two grey tubes for glucose measurement
  - Keep sample 4 labelled in the fridge for further potential tests or in case samples are lost
  - See page 229 for interpretation of lumbar puncture results

COMPLICATIONS

- Failure, difficulty locating space
- Post-dural puncture headache

- Nerve damage
- Infection
- Bleeding/haematoma

PEAK FLOW MONITORING AND INHALER TECHNIQUE

Over four million people in the UK have asthma. Inhalers are therefore widely used and correct technique is integral to dose delivery. Furthermore, peak expiratory flow rate (PEFR) measurement is an essential tool in diagnosing, monitoring and assessing severity of attacks.

PEAK EXPIRATORY FLOW RATE MONITORING

Most patients will be provided with their own peak flow meter. This will allow them to record morning and afternoon readings in a diary, to aid diagnosis (diurnal variation is often seen). It is recommended that this is done as follows:

- Stand up
- Put the marker to zero
- Take a deep breath
- Seal lips around meter mouthpiece
- Blow out as hard and fast as possible into the meter
- Note the value
- Repeat to a total of three times
- Record the highest reading
- Compare reading to a standard chart

PEFR is also used to assess effectiveness of inhalers, i.e. if performed before and after use.

INHALER TECHNIQUE

For metered-dose inhalers (MDIs)

- Stand up
- Shake inhaler before use and spray once into the air if not used for some time
- Take a few deep slow breaths and after breathing out place the MDI in your mouth, sealing the mouthpiece with your lips
- As you start to slowly breathe in, press down on the canister at the same time
- Hold your breath for up to 10 seconds, before breathing normally
- Repeat as directed

It is recommended that children should use a spacer device with their MDI. Children under the age of 3 may require a facemask, spacer and MDI. Children over the age of 7 may be able to use dry-powder or breath-actuated inhalers. Always check the child's inhaler technique or parent's administration technique.

SPACER TECHNIQUE

- Attach to a spacer device

- Place mouthpiece of spacer into mouth
- Child breathes in and out normally
- Squirt one puff every 10 seconds
- Can have up to 10 puffs in case of acute attack
- In mild–moderate attacks, an MDI and a spacer are as effective as a nebulizer

ACUTE TREATMENT

- β_2-agonists such as salbutamol are the mainstay of treatment in acute asthma
- They are known colloquially as 'relievers' and are MDIs that are usually blue

PREVENTER TREATMENT

- Steroid inhalers, such as beclometasone, are the mainstay of 'preventer' treatment
- They are usually supplied as brown or orange MDIs
- They need to be used regularly in order to be effective – usually one or two puffs in the morning and at bedtime
- It is important to wash out the mouth after use to prevent oral thrush
- The usual doses of inhaled steroids do not usually cause systemic side effects

SURGICAL HAND SCRUB AND GOWN

Surgical hand scrub and gown is a skill not only vital for assisting in theatre but also for undertaking sterile procedures such as central line and chest drain insertion.

INDICATIONS

- Invasive procedures:
  - Theatres: most surgical procedures
  - Sterile procedures: central line, chest drain insertion

CONTRAINDICATIONS

- Infected hand wounds – cuts should be covered with sterile dressing after scrub is performed

PREPARATION

- Ensure you:
  - Are wearing scrubs and appropriate theatre shoes
  - Have removed all jewellery and watches
  - Have short nails
  - Have a hat on with hair tucked in
  - Have a mask on with eye protection
- Assemble:
  - Sterile gown pack: open ensuring only the edges are touched to ensure sterile field created by opened pack is not contaminated
  - Sterile gloves (correct size): open and drop the sterile glove packet onto the open gown pack without touching it
  - Cleaning solution

TECHNIQUE

- Surgical handwashing should take at least 3 minutes using generous amounts of cleaning solution to form a lather
- Hands should be kept higher than elbows to avoid contaminated 'elbow water' dripping down towards the hands
- Turn the tap in the scrub sink on at a moderate flow
- Ensure the water is a comfortable temperature and wet arms from elbow to hands generously
- Select an elbow-operated antibacterial skin cleanser, e.g. chlorhexidine or povidone iodine
- Start with a 'social' handwash
- For the first scrub of the day take a new single use sterile brush with nail cleaner (repeated use is inadvisable as it may lead to damage to the skin and increased microbial colonization)
- After cleaning under every nail, apply cleaning solution to the brush and scrub your fingers, palm, back of hand and forearms to the elbow in that order
- Discard brush and nail cleaner in the sharps bin
- Rinse hands/forearms ensuring water flows from high hands to low elbows
- Reapply cleaning solution to hands and commence the following:
  - Start with palm to palm washing (Fig 3.5a)
  - Interlace the fingers (Fig 3.5b)
  - Place left palm over back of right hand and continue washing with fingers interlaced (Fig 3.5c)
  - Repeat with hands reversed
  - Rub the backs of the fingers of one hand in the palm of the other, with hands interlocked, and reverse
  - Grasp the right thumb in the palm of your left hand and rub in a circular fashion, and vice versa (Fig 3.5d)
  - Rub the fingers of the left hand in the palm of the right and vice versa (Fig 3.5e)
- The hands are now sterile and can only touch items within the sterile field created by the opened gown pack
- Dry with disposable towels found in gown pack – usually two, one for each hand
- Dry the hand thoroughly then wrist and finally forearm and dispose
- Repeat with new towel for other hand then wrist and forearm
- Don your gown, keeping it over your hands as much as possible
- Ask an assistant to tie the gown up from behind
- Don your gloves (consider two pairs in high-risk procedures)
- Take paper tab, holding both ends of gown belt, and release left hand gown belt from tab, keeping hold of it in your right hand
- Hand the tab to an assistant and allow them to come around you to wrap the belt
- Re-take the right hand portion of the belt in your right hand firmly without touching the tab, which is now unsterile, and allow your assistant to pull the tab off
- Tie the belt in a double bow on your left side
- Keep your hands within the sterile field or folded across your chest

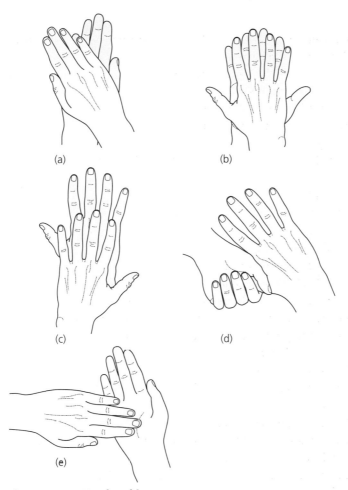

Figure 3.5a–e Handwashing

COMPLICATIONS

- Allergy – latex gloves/cleaning solution
  - ○ Latex free sterile gloves available
  - ○ Use alternative cleaning solution if allergic
- Irritation and dry skin (moisturize, moisturize, moisturize!)
- Contamination of surgical field if scrub technique improperly performed

SIMPLE SUTURING

Outside the operating theatre suturing is used by doctors and specialist nurses for simple procedures and injuries.

INDICATIONS

- Procedures, e.g. suturing in chest drains and central lines
- Superficial wound closure (e.g. in the Accident and Emergency setting)

It is important to note that only certain wounds are appropriate for primary closure by a non-surgeon.

CONTRAINDICATIONS

- Patient refusal despite careful explanation of risks and benefits
- Large, complicated wounds
- Foreign body in wounds
- Local infection

PREPARATION

- Obtain consent
- Explain procedure
- Assemble:
    - Sterile pack and gauze
    - Needle-holder
    - Traumatic (toothed) forceps (for handling skin when suturing)
    - Atraumatic (non-toothed) forceps (for preventing puncture when handling delicate structures such as bowel or arteries)
    - Appropriate suture (see Box 3.5)
    - Cleaning solution, e.g. sterile saline
    - Dressing
    - Sterile gloves

BOX 3.5 RECOMMENDED SUTURE MATERIALS

Non-absorbable, monofilaments, e.g. Prolene

Site	Size	Removal
Face laceration	5–0 to 6–0	~5 days
Scalp and chest	4–0	~10 days
Limbs and abdomen	4–0	~10 days

POSITIONING

- As best to allow comfort for patient and expose wound optimally

SOLUTION

- Use 1 per cent or 2 per cent lidocaine to anaesthetize the area

TECHNIQUE

- Explain the procedure
- Gain informed consent
- Remove all clothing or jewellery from below the elbow and don sterile gloves
- Clean the wound adopting an aseptic technique
- Drape the area around the wound to ensure a sterile field
- Infiltrate with 2–10 mL of 1 per cent or 2 per cent lidocaine (depending on size of wound) and allow it to work for 5 minutes

- Select the appropriate suture material (depending on site)
- Grip the needle with the needle-holder two-thirds of the way from the point (Fig 3.6a)
- Start your first suture in the middle of a wound and the second in the middle on the remaining wound and so on
- Insert the needle into the skin 5–10 mm from the wound edge, perpendicularly at a position to gain an optimal 'bite' (Fig 3.6b)
- Retrieve the needle from the middle of the wound with traumatic forceps
- Re-enter the other side of the wound, exiting the skin at a distance identical to the other side (Fig 3.6c)
- Pull the suture through the wound by the suture itself, leaving enough to tie a knot (Fig 3.6d)
- Lie the needle-holder across the length of wound and turn the longer length (attached to needle) of suture around it twice and pull the first throw tight (Fig 3.6e and f)
- Repeat a single throw back over the wound (Fig 3.6g)
- Repeat a final throw in the original direction (Fig 3.6h)
- Pull the finished knot to one side of the wound and cut the ends at roughly 1 cm (Fig 3.6i)
- Repeat for the remaining sutures until wound edges are neatly opposed – do not place the sutures so tightly that the wound is under tension
- Cover with a dressing and provide patient with appropriate information for looking after wound and suture removal

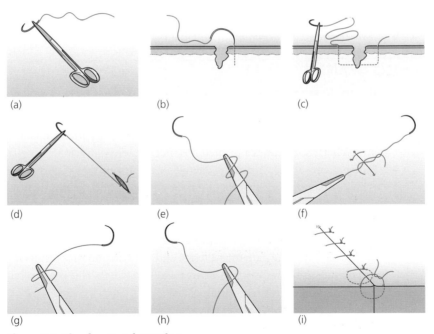

(a)   (b)   (c)

(d)   (e)   (f)

(g)   (h)   (i)

Figure 3.6 Simple wound suturing

> **BOX 3.6 TYPES OF SUTURING**
>
> - Interrupted (as above) – ideal for simple skin/subcutaneous tissue wounds
> - Continuous subcuticular – for surgical wound providing good aesthetic effect, absorbable or non-absorbable sutures may be used
> - Mattress – for wounds likely to be under tension, e.g. natal cleft

COMPLICATIONS

- Wound dehiscence
- Infection
- Haematoma, bleeding

WRITING A DRUG CHART

From day 1, all junior doctors are required to prescribe a large array of medications. Despite being an everyday occurrence, mistakes can be easily made and the consequences can be serious.

PREPARATION

- Drug prescription chart
- Black ink pen with water resistant ink
- *British National Formulary* or hospital formulary (if required)

TECHNIQUE

Drug prescription charts vary from hospital to hospital. The following is a guide to what will be required on the front of most charts.

- The name, date of birth and hospital number of the patient must be printed on the drug chart. Sometimes a printed hospital sticker is sufficient
- The patient's weight – noting if actual or estimated
- The number of drug charts in total for a patient, and the number of a particular chart within that total (e.g. II of III, for the second chart in a set of three)
- The ward on which the patient is based
- The name or initials of the consultant under whose care the patient is
- Drugs to which the patient is allergic and the reaction that results if the patient is exposed (e.g. erythromycin – nausea and vomiting). This is often required to be visible on each page of the prescription chart
- The date the chart has been created

BOX 3.7 FILLING IN DRUG CHARTS

Most charts will have different sections to accommodate different dosing schedules:

- Once-only drugs, for example pre-procedure sedation with midazolam
- Drugs that can be given as required, such as an antiemetic if the patient develops nausea
- Variable-dose drugs, such as a chlordiazepoxide reducing regimen for alcohol withdrawal
- Regular drugs to be given at a fixed time every day, e.g. antihypertensives
- Intravenous fluids and infusions
- There may be a separate chart for insulin, warfarin, and infusions such as heparin

---

All drugs have very specific prescription criteria, and must be written clearly with:

- Drug name – printed (generic name preferred)
- Dose and units written legibly (some charts may have units printed that you can circle to limit the possibility of dosing errors). It is generally better to write the whole word than the abbreviation (micrograms, rather than μg or mcg)
- Route of administration – either oral (per os), intravenous (iv), intramuscular (im), subcutaneous (sc), nebulized (neb), inhaled (inh), topical (top) – and specify site
- Frequency – once daily (od) twice daily (bd) etc
- Prescriber's surname – printed
- Prescriber's signature
- Prescriber's grade (e.g. FY1)
- Prescriber's bleep number (or similar contact number for queries)
- Time prescribed (for one-off drugs)
- Time to be given (for regular drugs – try to prescribe at times that the nursing staff do their drug administration rounds)
- The length of course. This can often be written in a 'notes' box, or similar and is useful in, for example, the prescription of antibiotics

When crossing off a drug you should:

- Put a single wavy line through the prescription – but do not obliterate any of the details – they may be useful when reviewing the patient later during the admission
- Put two vertical parallel lines at the end of the last dose you want to be given
- Sign and date the crossed-off row and write the word 'STOPPED' on the chart

Follow-up:

- All new prescriptions should be documented in the patient's notes with doses, route of administration, length of course and reason for commencing the drug
- If a drug is stopped, document this in the patient's notes with the reason why. If it is due to an allergic reaction, add it to the allergies box on the chart as well
- If unsure about a drug dose or route of administration check in the *British National Formulary*, which should be available on every ward or online (www.bnf.org.uk). It can also be used to check for indications, potential side effects, interactions and contraindications. There are also specific appendices for the use of drugs in liver disease, renal impairment, pregnancy and breastfeeding

- If a drug dose is changed it is good practice to rewrite the whole drug prescription, not simply cross out the old dose and write in the new one

COMPLICATIONS

Mistakes are usually due to a lack of care when prescribing. A busy junior doctor must take the time to ensure that they do not accidentally:

- Prescribe the wrong drug, especially when they look or sound similar (e.g. chlorpromazine/carbamazepine) or write illegibly so the incorrect drug is administered
- Prescribe the wrong units, e.g. micrograms versus milligrams
- Prescribe the units ambiguously – 10 iu (international units) may be read as 101 u (units), leading to a massive overdose
- Write the wrong route, e.g. an oral fluid given intravenously
- Miscalculate the dose, particularly relevant in paediatrics, where drug doses are often weight dependent
- Fail to clearly cross off a drug so it continues to be given
- Prescribe once-weekly drugs so they are given daily
- Prescribe the same drug and dose via different routes when in fact the dose should change depending on route, e.g. morphine
- Miss a drug interaction

Note

A few drugs, predominantly those that are modified-release preparations, should be prescribed by their brand name as their performance characteristics may vary.

INTRAVENOUS DRUG ADMINISTRATION

INDICATIONS

- Drugs altered or not absorbed by the gastrointestinal tract effectively
- Rapid therapeutic effect required
- The patient is not able to take oral medication

CONTRAINDICATIONS

- Patient refusal despite careful explanation of risks and benefits
- No venous access

PREPARATION

- Explain procedure
- Obtain consent
- Assemble:
  - Prescription chart with the drug correctly prescribed
  - Alcohol gel for cleaning hands
  - Disposable tray
  - Gloves
  - Alcohol swabs

○ Correct drug vial and dosage
○ Dilutant (e.g. sterile water for injection or normal saline), needle and syringe
○ Two saline flushes with drawing-up needle and 10 mL syringe
○ Sharps bin
○ Drug label

POSITIONING

● Sit patient comfortably and ensure easy access to cannula site

TECHNIQUE

● Ensure the drug is correctly prescribed for the correct patient
● Check allergy status
● Wash hands and don gloves
● Draw up two saline flushes
● Check the drug dosage and expiry date of the drug and dilutant
● Double check the drug, dilutant and saline with a qualified person and get them to sign the drug chart
● Draw up the correct amount of dilutant for the drug using a needle and syringe
● Flip the cap off the drug vial and clean with a swab, allow to dry and then pierce the vial and add the dilutant, holding the plunger on the syringe depressed
● Shake until the drug is fully dissolved
● Holding the vial upside down, release the plunger of the syringe when the needle is below the fluid level. This will allow the drug solution to fill the syringe until the vial is empty
● Label the syringe
● Dispose of any needles into a sharps bin
● Take the drug and drug chart to the bedside
● Check the patient's details (using wrist band, drug chart and verbally) and gain informed consent
● Check the cannula site for any signs of infection and date of insertion
● Clean the cannula injection port with alcohol swab and leave to dry
● Flush the cannula with saline
● Administer the drug at the recommended rate, initially 1 mL, observing for any local or systemic reactions
● Flush the cannula with saline at the end of drug administration
● Inform the patient of any symptoms they may experience
● Dispose of the equipment correctly
● Wash hands
● Follow-up:
  ○ Sign, date and document the time on the drug chart
  ○ Fill in a yellow card if a serious adverse reaction occurs
  ○ Inform a senior immediately if a drug error or adverse reaction occurs

COMPLICATIONS

● Local reaction to drug/phlebitis
● Side effects of medication

- Anaphylaxis
- Drug error

BLOOD TRANSFUSION

INDICATIONS

- Symptomatic anaemia
- Acute blood loss (e.g. variceal bleed)
- Intra- and postoperative blood replacement
- Before radiotherapy: haemoglobin should be >10 g/dL

CONTRAINDICATIONS

Absolute

- Patient refusal (e.g. for reasons of religious beliefs regarding the use of blood products as in Jehovah's Witnesses), despite careful explanation of risks and benefits

Relative

- Previous transfusion reaction (this does not mean a necessary transfusion should not be administered, but care should be taken when cross-matching and infusing the products)

PREPARATION

Obtaining a cross-match sample

- Explain the need for a blood transfusion and obtain informed verbal consent
- Confirm the patient's details with them and their name tag
- Perform phlebotomy (see p. 172)
- Clearly complete the patient's details *by hand* on the blood bottle at the bedside after drawing blood
- Complete the transfusion request form:
  - Write the patient's details as on the bottle
  - Sign and print your name clearly and add your contact details, along with the consultant's name
  - Clearly describe what products you would like (and the quantity and desired date and time)
  - Document the reason for the request
    - Certain surgical procedures will have the number of units of blood pre-decided by the trust
  - Other non-essential, but useful, information for the laboratory includes previous pregnancy, ethnic origin and previous transfusions

Laboratory tests

- All samples are ABO and rhesus D typed in the laboratory, along with an antibody screen
- If red cell antibodies are detected then full identification of these is performed

- In certain situations, e.g. in immunocompromised patients following bone marrow transplantation, more specific blood products, such as cytomegalovirus negative and irradiated, will be required

TECHNIQUE

- Ensure the correct blood products are clearly prescribed on the patient's drug chart, with the correct date, time and infusion details
- Carefully inspect the blood bag for discoloration, clots and leaks
- Reconfirm the patient's details with them, their name bracelet and ensure they are identical to those on the drug chart
- The products will be supplied with a (pink) printed form from the blood bank with the patient's details and corresponding unit codes (and expiry dates) on it
- With another healthcare professional confirm:
  - The patient information is correct
  - The units numbers, blood type and expiry date listed on the printed form match those on the bags
- Both professionals should sign the printed form to confirm the blood has been checked and is ready to transfuse
- If you identify any inconsistencies with any of the above data, the transfusion must *not* be given
- The above information is rechecked at the patient bedside just prior to administration of the product
- A set of baseline observations should be performed prior to the commencement of the infusion (see p. 167)
- Document the date and time of administration, the serial code of the blood bag used and sign and print your name

INFUSION

- Specially designed giving sets, with slightly different filters, are available for different blood product transfusions
- Red blood cells must be commenced within 30 minutes of their removal from the refrigerator and should not be left hanging for more than 4 hours
- Platelets must be used within 1 hour of issue
- Fresh frozen plasma should be used within 24 hours of thawing
- Blood products can be given via any size cannula, though this will determine the speed at which it can be administered. The recommended minimum is 18 gauge

FOLLOW-UP

- Observations should be performed regularly during the transfusion
- The observer should be vigilant for signs of a transfusion reaction, and if any of these are displayed the transfusion should be stopped
- Following a transfusion the patient can develop new antibodies to red cells and if another transfusion is required after 48–72 hours a fresh group and save will be required

COMPLICATIONS

- Adverse reactions to a blood transfusion are not uncommon
- They can be acute (within 24 hours), or delayed (>24 hours) and mild, moderate or severe (life threatening)
- Symptoms and signs range from fever, rash, muscle pains, agitation and tachycardia to hypotension and shock
- The primary management is to stop the transfusion immediately and perform a complete assessment of the patient including rechecking the match between the patient and the blood product
- Long-term complications include the transmission of blood-borne viruses such as hepatitis B or C and human immunodeficiency virus. Although greatly reduced with careful donor selection and rigorous sample testing, this is still a small but real risk

Emergencies

BASIC LIFE SUPPORT

ALGORITHM

Check it is: **SAFE TO APPROACH**

Is the patient: **UNRESPONSIVE**

If so: **SHOUT FOR HELP**

And: **OPEN AIRWAY**
Head tilt, chin lift (and jaw thrust for non-lay rescuers)
Clear any easy-to-remove airway obstruction

Assess: **BREATHING**
LOOK for chest movement, LISTEN for breath sounds
FEEL for air on your cheek and chest expansion, for 10 seconds.

No breathing: **CALL 999**

Start: **CHEST COMPRESSIONS**
Place heel of your hand over lower third of sternum, place the heel of your other hand over it and interlock fingers
Aim to achieve depression of sternum – 4–5 cm
Ratio of 2 breaths to 30 compressions
Rate of 100/min

If another rescuer is present alternate who does cardiopulmonary resuscitation (CPR) every 2 minutes to prevent fatigue

One rescuer should perform breaths, while the other performs compression

If breaths are ineffective, with airway manoeuvres, or the rescuers are unwilling, continue with chest compressions alone

Ref: Resuscitation Council guidelines

FOREIGN BODY AIRWAY OBSTRUCTION

- This typically presents as a sudden onset of coughing, gagging or stridor and respiratory distress
- Assess severity

Effective cough

- Encourage coughing and monitor for deterioration or expectoration of foreign body

Ineffective cough

- Conscious but shows signs of airway obstruction
  - ○ Stand to the side and slightly behind the victim
  - ○ Support the patient with one hand and lean them as far forwards as possible
  - ○ Give up to 5 sharp back blows, between the shoulder blades, with the heel of your hand
- If no response to back blows, try Heimlich's manoeuvre:
  - ○ Stand behind patient with arms around the upper abdomen
  - ○ Clench fist between the umbilicus and xiphisternum
  - ○ Pull sharply upwards and inwards giving up to 5 thrusts
- Unconscious
  - ○ Give 5 breaths
  - ○ Commence CPR

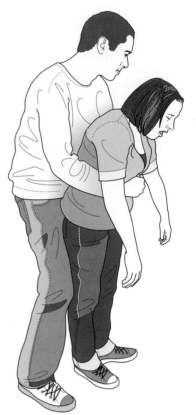

Figure 4.1 Heimlich's manoeuvre

AIRWAY MANAGEMENT

Basic airway management is a potentially life-saving skill that all doctors should be skilled in. It is the first system to be addressed when assessing an unwell patient.

INITIAL ASSESSMENT

Initial airway assessment should include:

- Looking in the mouth for any obvious or easy to retrieve foreign bodies, e.g. dentures, that could be contributing to any airway obstruction
- Careful suctioning under direct vision may be employed at this point

AIRWAY MANOEUVRES

There are three basic airway manoeuvres that can be employed in an unstable patient. They are:

- Head tilt – the head is tipped upwards to the 'sniffing the morning air' position (note this is *not* appropriate for patients you believe may have sustained a cervical spine injury)
- Chin lift – the chin is pulled up towards the ceiling
- Jaw thrust – fingers are placed bilaterally behind the angle of the jaw, again thrusting it towards the ceiling

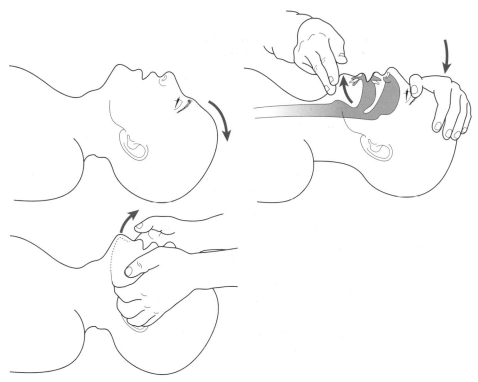

Figure 4.2 Airway manoeuvres: head tilt, chin lift, jaw thrust

Airway adjuncts

Once the airway is clear and the above manoeuvres have been employed, airway adjuncts can be used.

- Nasopharyngeal airway:
    - Inserted via the nostril into the nasopharynx
    - Sized by selecting one that is similar to the dimensions of the patient's little finger
    - Lubricate well with aqueous jelly
    - Ensure a safety pin is inserted through the nasal end, to prevent it being swallowed or aspirated

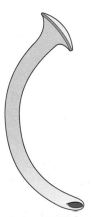

Figure 4.3 Nasopharyngeal airway

- Oropharyngeal airway (Guedel airway)
  - These C-shaped reinforced airways are best tolerated in patients with decreased consciousness
  - It is sized by selecting the one that corresponds best to the distance between the angle of the jaw to the incisors.
  - They are inserted upside-down and then turned back to their formal position

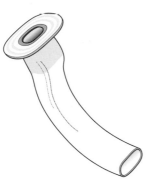

Figure 4.4 Guedel airway

Both these adjuncts should be used with 15 L of oxygen via a non-rebreathing facemask.

If the patient is making no, or inadequate, respiratory effort a bag-valve-mask device can be used to hand ventilate the patient.

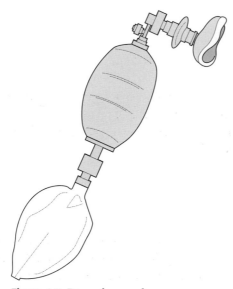

Figure 4.5 Bag-valve-mask

ADVANCED AIRWAY MANAGEMENT

If ventilation is inadequate with the above interventions then more advanced adjuncts can be used by an airways expert, e.g. an anaesthetist.

Laryngeal mask airway:

- This device is easy to insert and is an alternative to bag-valve-mask ventilation
- Most women take a size 3 or 4, most men a size 4 or 5
- It is inserted into the oropharynx, after lubrication until it meets resistance

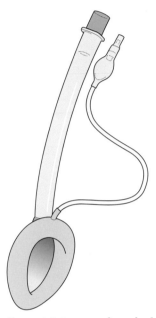

Figure 4.6 Laryngeal mask airway

Endotracheal tube:

- This can only be inserted by those trained to do so
- It involves the use of a laryngoscope
- Once inserted, and the cuff inflated within the trachea, this constitutes a secure airway and protects against aspiration of gastric contents
- Ventilation via an endotracheal tube can occur simultaneously with chest compressions, without the need for pauses

GLASGOW COMA SCALE

There are several ways in which to assess the conscious level of a patient. The Glasgow Coma Scale (GCS) has been adopted as the gold standard in hospitals throughout the world. It is not, however, a substitute for a formal neurological examination, which should be done at the same time.

Patients are assessed according to their eye opening (scores 1–4), verbal response (scores 1–5) and motor response (scores 1–6): 15 is the maximum, 3 is the lowest. It is essential that the patient's *best* response is recorded.

Response to painful stimuli is best assessed centrally, such as pressure on supraorbital ridges or trapezius muscle.

EYE OPENING

- Eyes open spontaneously – 4
- Eyes open to voice – 3
- Eyes open to pain – 2
- Eyes not opening – 1

VERBAL RESPONSE

- Normal, orientated speech – 5
- Disorientated speech – 4
- Inappropriate words – 3
- Incomprehensible sounds – 2
- No sounds made – 1

MOTOR RESPONSE

- Obeys commands – 6
- Localises to painful stimuli – 5
- Flexion withdrawal to painful stimuli – 4
- Abnormal flexion to painful stimuli – 3
- Extends to painful stimuli – 2
- No response – 1

ALTERNATIVE METHODS

It is acceptable to use 'AVPU' to rapidly classify levels of consciousness in some situations.

- A – alert
- V – responds to verbal stimuli
- P – responds to painful stimuli
- U – unresponsive

Interpretations

ELECTROCARDIOGRAMS

A systematic approach to the ECG is essential so that all abnormalities can be detected and the underlying cardiac activity, even in unusual ECGs, deduced.

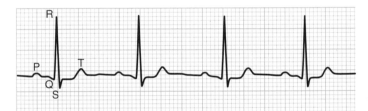

Figure 5.1 Normal electrocardiogram (ECG)

PATIENT DETAILS

- State the patient's name, age and date on which ECG was taken
- State whether any chest pain was recorded at that time

RATE

- At standard paper speed (25 mm/s) each small square on the ECG represents 0.04 seconds (1/25th second)
- Calculate the rate by counting the number of large squares between two consecutive R waves and dividing 300 by this number
- Normal heart rate for adults is defined as 60–100 beats/min

RHYTHM

- Assess whether the rhythm is sinus i.e. each QRS complex is preceded by a P wave
- Regular
- Irregular:
  - Irregularly irregular, i.e. atrial fibrillation
  - Regularly irregular, e.g. second-degree heart block

AXIS

- This represents the mean electrical vector of the heart
- Normal axis is −30 to +90°
- The simplest way to determine the axis is to look at leads I and AVF
  - Lead I and AVF both positive: normal axis (SE quadrant)
  - Lead I and AVF both negative: 'northwest territory'
  - Lead I negative and AVF positive: right axis deviation (SW quadrant)
  - Lead I positive and AVF negative: 'left' (NE) quadrant
    - If lead II is positive in this case: normal axis
    - If lead II is negative: left axis deviation.

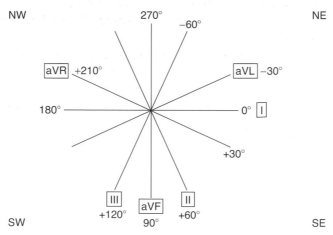

Figure 5.2 The cardiac axis

P WAVE

- The P wave represents atrial depolarization
- It should be less than 2.5 mm (2.5 small squares) high and 0.08 ms (2 small squares) wide
- Abnormalities include:
  - Absent: atrial fibrillation (no organized atrial contraction)
  - Bifid p waves: 'p mitrale' – left atrial hypertrophy
  - Tall p waves: 'p pulmonale' – right atrial hypertrophy

PR INTERVAL

- The PR interval is measured from the *beginning* of the P wave to the beginning of the QRS complex
- The normal value of the PR interval is 0.12–0.2 seconds (3–5 small squares)
- A prolonged PR interval is caused by a delay in conduction from the sinoatrial (SA) node to the atrioventricular (AV) node, seen in:
  - First-degree heart block
  - Electrolyte disturbances (e.g. hyper/hypokalaemia)
- A short PR interval is seen if there is abnormal conduction tissue between the atrium and the ventricles (e.g. Wolff–Parkinson–White syndrome)

QRS COMPLEX

- The QRS complex is created by the depolarization of the ventricle
- It should be no wider than 0.12 seconds (3 small squares)
- Anything broader than this suggests a disruption in the usual efficient depolarization, for example bundle branch block
- A normal QRS complex is up to 30 mm high, although in some young thin men it may be taller.

ST SEGMENTS

- The ST segment runs from where the QRS complex finishes to where the T wave starts
- It should be in the same plane as the baseline – isoelectric
- An ST segment more than 0.5 mm below the baseline is considered depressed, indicating myocardial ischaemia
- An ST segment elevated more than 1 mm above the baseline can be caused by:
  - Myocardial ischaemia, e.g. myocardial infarction
  - Pericarditis
  - Normal finding, e.g. 'high take-off' or benign repolarization, normal in young Afro-Caribbean patients
- The shape of the ST segment, with clinical correlation, can help differentiate this

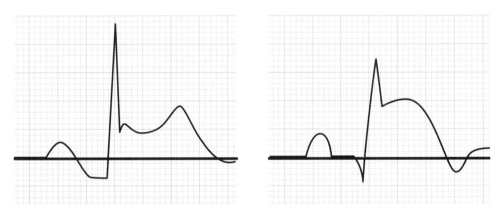

Figure 5.3 ST elevation: (a) pericarditis and (b) myocardial infarction

T WAVE

- The T wave is produced by ventricular repolarization
- It should be round, upright and convex, except in leads aVR, III and sometimes V1 or V2 where it may be inverted
- Abnormal T wave inversion is a non-specific sign of ischaemia
- Tall or peaked T waves are seen in hyperkalaemia (see below) or acute myocardial injury

COMMON ECG PATTERNS
Atrial fibrillation

- Disorganized atrial activity
- Absent P waves
- Irregularly irregular rhythm

- Narrow QRS complexes

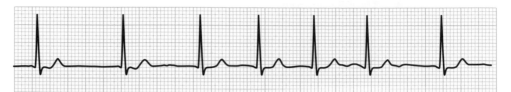

Figure 5.4 Atrial fibrillation

Ventricular tachycardia

- Wide, regular, bizarrely shaped QRS complexes
- May or may not be associated with a cardiac output
- Very unstable rhythm – may deteriorate to ventricular fibrillation or asystole if not treated
- *Cardiac arrest rhythm – requires emergency treatment/defibrillation*

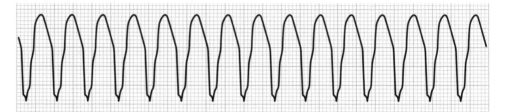

Figure 5.5 Ventricular tachycardia

Ventricular fibrillation

- Chaotic ECG
- No recognizable pattern
- *Cardiac arrest rhythm – requires emergency treatment/defibrillation*
- **Note:** Check rhythm in all leads

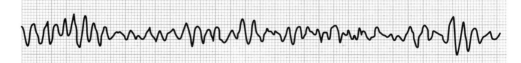

Figure 5.6 Ventricular fibrillation

Asystole

- Incompatible with life
- No electrical activity from heart
- *Cardiac arrest rhythm – requires emergency treatment*
- **Note:** Make sure all leads are attached

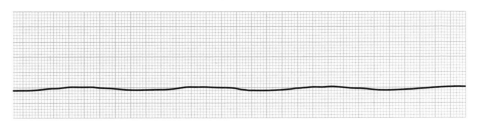

Figure 5.7 ECG: Asystole

Hyperkalaemia

- Tall or 'tented' T waves
- Flattened (or absent) P waves
- Prolonged PR interval
- Broad QRS complex
- Arrhythmias (increased chance if $K^+ > 7$)

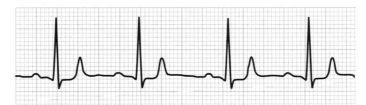

Figure 5.8 ECG: Hyperkalaemia

Atrial flutter

- Tachycardia due to re-entrant circuit in the atrium
- Characteristic 'saw-tooth' baseline
- Atrial rate usually approximately 300 beats/min
- Ventricular rate usually approximately 150 beats/min (in 2:1 block)

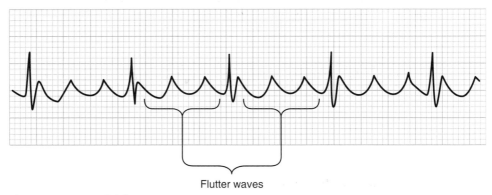

Flutter waves

Figure 5.9 ECG: Atrial flutter

Myocardial infarction

- ST elevation in leads representing area affected by infarction
- ST depression in reciprocal leads
- Pathological Q waves
- T wave inversion

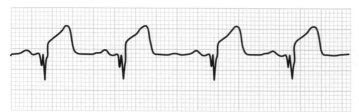

Figure 5.10 ECG: Myocardial infarction

Table 5.1 Localizing the site of a myocardial infarction

Location of infarction	ECG leads affected	Artery affected
Inferior	ST elevation >1 mm in two or more of leads II, III, AVF	Right coronary
Anterior	ST elevation >2 mm in two or more adjacent leads V2, V3, V4	Left anterior descending (LAD)
Anteroseptal	ST elevation >2 mm in two or more adjacent leads V1, V2, V3	LAD
Lateral	ST elevation >2 mm in two or more adjacent leads V5, V6, I, AVL	Circumflex

Atrioventricular (heart) block

- First-degree block – prolonged PR interval (>0.2 seconds – 5 small squares)
- Second-degree block:
    - Mobitz type I (Wenckebach) – progressive elongation of PR interval until a P wave is 'dropped'
    - Mobitz type II – normal PR interval, interspersed with blocked P waves. May exhibit, e.g. 2:1, 3:1 block.
- Third-degree block – complete heart block. Displays P wave activity with no discernable relationship to the QRS complexes

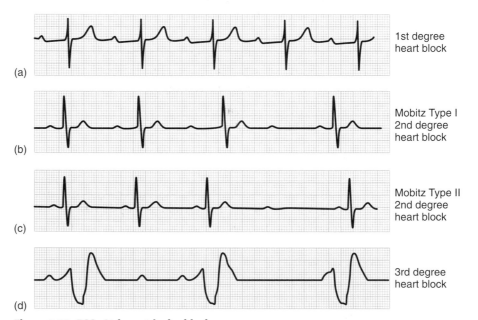

Figure 5.11 ECG: Atrioventricular block

CHEST X-RAY

The chest X-ray is a useful, cheap and effective method of imaging the chest.

EXAMINING A FILM

It is important to take a systematic approach to interpreting the chest X-ray. A suggested methodical way to present it is as follows:

- 'This is a plain PA [posteroanterior]/AP [anteroposterior] chest X-ray of (patients name and age)'
- Comment on the film quality:
  - Penetration: good contrast between 'black and white' areas, are the vertebral bodies visible behind the heart?
  - Rotation: are the medial heads of the clavicles central with respect to the spinous processes?
- Lung fields – compare right to left:
  - Size
  - Lucency
  - Focal shadowing
- Heart – examine for:
  - Dextrocardia (check the marker placed by the radiographer)
  - Heart size – the maximum width of the heart should be less than half the width of the total thoracic cavity (an AP view will artificially enlarge the heart size, making it difficult to comment)
  - Outline of the cardiac borders
- Mediastinum:
  - Position of the trachea – any deviation
  - The aortic knuckle will be visible as a semicircle above the left heart border
- Bones:
  - Fractures, e.g. causing pneumothorax, haemothorax
  - Bony metastases, e.g. breast cancer (mastectomy may also be visible)
  - Missing ribs, e.g. from a thoracotomy
- Soft tissues:
  - Symmetry
  - Normal breast shadows
- Hemidiaphragm:
  - Convex, smooth
  - Costophrenic angles – blunting: effusions, pleural thickening, consolidation
  - Normal gastric bubble (under left hemidiaphragm)
  - Abnormal air under the diaphragm (e.g. gastric perforation)

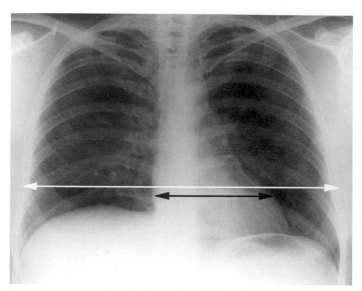

Figure 5.12 Measuring the heart size: divide the size of the heart (black arrow) by the width of the thorax (white arrow). A normal value is less than 0.5

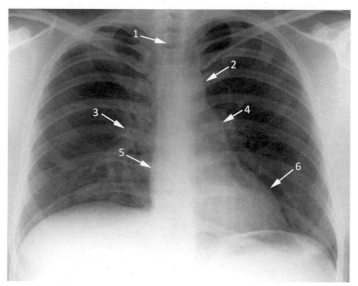

Figure 5.13 Normal landmarks on posteroanterior chest X-ray. 1 – trachea; 2 – aortic knuckle formed by the aortic arch; 3 – right hilum; 4 – left hilum; 5 – pulmonary artery; 6 – left atrium

COMMON EXAM X-RAYS
Consolidation

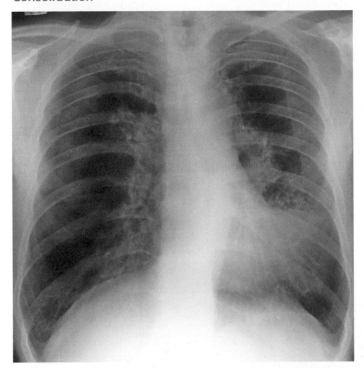

Figure 5.14 Pneumonia with consolidation of the lingula – loss of the left heart border

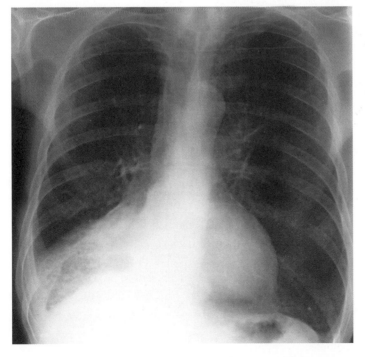

Figure 5.15 Right lobar pneumonia with air bronchogram

Consolidation is caused by air space shadowing and appears as an area of ill-defined opacification within the lung spaces. Within the area of consolidation air bronchograms are seen as the black outlines of air-filled bronchi contrasting against the fluid-filled airspaces.

Common causes include:

- Infection (lobar pneumonia)
- Pulmonary infarction
- Pus
- Aspiration pneumonia or atypical pneumonia, e.g. *Pneumocystis jirovecii* (bilateral consolidation), previously called PCP

Note: Consolidation can be difficult to distinguish from collapse.

Collapse exhibits:

- A well-defined area of opacification with straight edges
- Distortion of the other anatomical markers as the lung volume shrinks
- Elevation of hemidiaphragm on the ipsilateral side

Pleural effusion

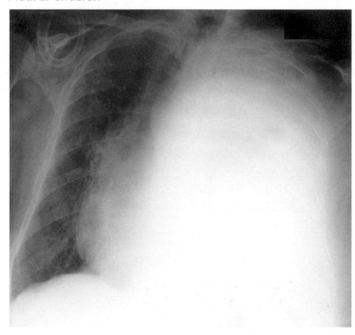

Figure 5.16 Opaque left hemithorax due to a large left pleural effusion

- An effusion appears as homogeneous shadowing, often with a curved upper border (meniscus)
- Small effusions may be seen as blunting of the costophrenic angle
- There must be at least 300 mL of fluid present to be seen on chest X-ray.
- Effusions can be caused by any fluid, which are indistinguishable on an X-ray (see p. 230)
    - Transudate
    - Exudate
    - Blood
    - Pus
    - Lymph

Single pulmonary mass

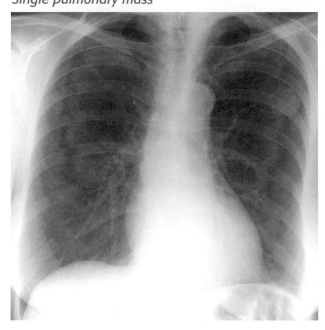

Figure 5.17 Left peripheral bronchial carcinoma

When a solitary pulmonary mass is seen on X-ray, malignancy must be excluded. Primary bronchial carcinomas are often round or spiculated and usually greater than 3 cm in size.

The differential diagnosis includes:

- A solitary metastasis
- Tuberculoma (usually calcified)
- Benign bronchial adenoma or hamartoma
- Abscess (often cavitating)
- Hydatid cyst (often cavitating)

Multiple pulmonary masses

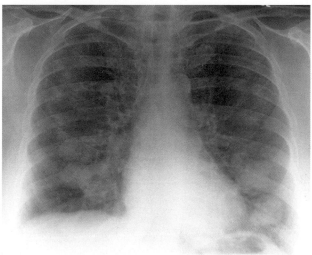

Figure 5.18 Multiple 'cannon ball' metastases from renal cell cancer

The differential diagnosis includes:

- Pulmonary metastases (common primaries: kidney, breast, thyroid)
- Rheumatoid nodules*
- Abscesses (often *Staphylococcus aureus*)*
- Wegener's granulomatosis*
- Caplan's syndrome* – pneumoconiosis and rheumatoid arthritis
- Hydatid cysts*

*May be cavitating.

Heart failure

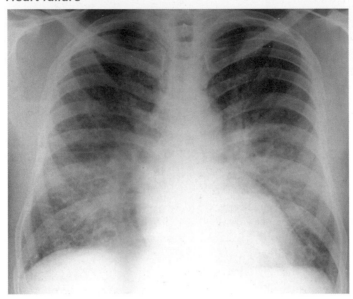

Figure 5.19 Acute left ventricular failure

Features of acute left ventricular failure:

- Upper lobe diversion: prominent upper lobe pulmonary vasculature
- 'Bat's wings' hilar shadowing: alveolar shadowing caused by pulmonary oedema
- Kerley B lines: small lines at the periphery of the lung field caused by interstitial oedema
- Enlarged heart: suggesting chronic heart failure

PNEUMOTHORAX

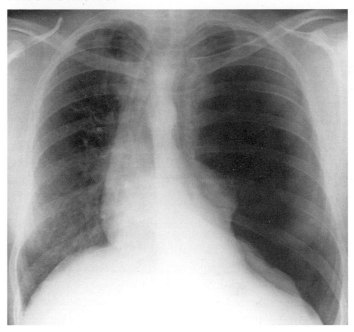

Figure 5.20 Left tension pneumothorax with midline shift. Note the mediastinal shift away from the affected side

Appearances on X-ray:

- Small pneumothorax: a black rim of air is seen surrounding the lung edge
- Large pneumothorax: affected lung field may be completely black and the lung collapsed down towards the mediastinum
- Tension pneumothorax: mediastinum is shifted away from the side of the pneumothorax – this requires urgent needle decompression

INTERSTITIAL LUNG DISEASE

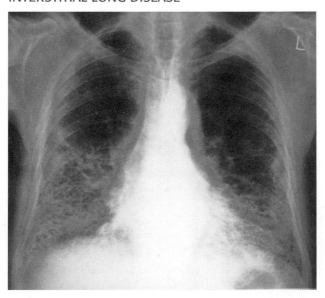

Figure 5.21 Basal lung fibrosis: reticular shadowing at the bases with sparing of the upper zones. Note the loss of the cardiac outline from the adjacent fibrosis

Long standing fibrotic changes appear as reticular (net-like) shadowing in both lung fields.

Causes include:

- Inorganic substances (asbestosis, silicosis)
- Drug induced (nitrofurantoin, bleomycin, amiodarone, methotrexate)
- Connective tissue diseases (rheumatoid arthritis, systemic sclerosis, systemic lupus erythematosus)
- Sarcoidosis
- Idiopathic
- Malignancy (lymphangitic carcinomatosis)

ABDOMINAL X-RAY

Abdominal X-rays can be an important part of the investigation of patients with abdominal pain. However, they should only be performed when the X-ray will provide important information in relation to a suspected diagnosis.

EXAMINING A FILM

It is important to take a systematic approach to interpreting the abdominal X-ray and to present it as follows:

- 'This is a supine [decubitus] or erect abdominal X-ray of [patient's name and age]'
- Gas pattern – look for:
  - The distribution of intraluminal gas shadowing (air inside the bowel).
  - Extraluminal gas – this is abnormal and indicates either a perforated viscus or recent surgery (e.g. laparoscopic)
- Small bowel: loops are centrally placed and have bands known as valvulae conniventes running across the bowel. Maximum diameter – 3.5 cm
- Large bowel: peripherally positioned, has mucosal folds which only partly span the width of the bowel wall (haustrae). Maximum diameter – 5 cm
- Calcification:
  - Check for any bony abnormalities, e.g. Paget's diseases, sacroiliitis or bone metastases
  - If abnormal calcification is seen it is important to identify the position of the opacity and relate it to the anatomy (see below)

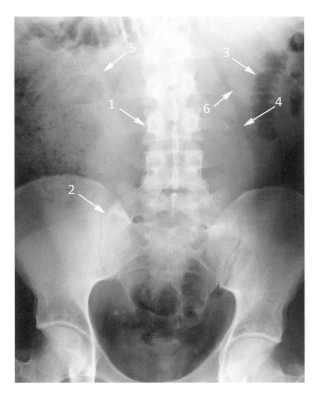

Figure 5.22 Anatomical landmarks on normal abdominal X-ray. 1 – lumbar spine; 2 – sacroiliac joints; 3 – gas in bowel; 4 – psoas shadow; 5 – right kidney; 6 – left kidney

SMALL BOWEL OBSTRUCTION

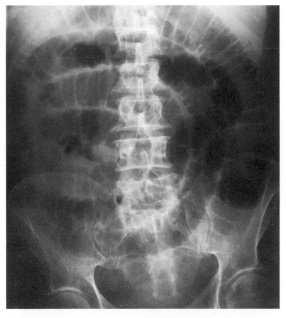

Figure 5.23 Small bowel obstruction

Features:

- Multiple dilated small bowel loops clustered in the centre of the film
- Thin valvulae conniventes seen passing across the lumen
- Air–fluid levels in the erect view
- Common causes: adhesions, hernias, gallstones (rare), intraluminal tumours (rare)

VOLVULUS AND LARGE BOWEL OBSTRUCTION

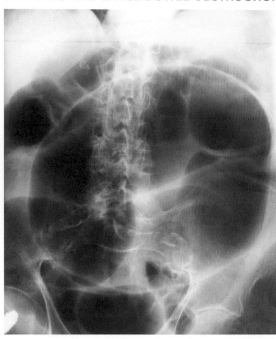

Figure 5.24 Sigmoid volvulus with 'coffee bean' sign

Features:

- A double loop of markedly distended large bowel caused by twisting of the bowel on itself and causing obstruction
- Often occurs at sigmoid but can occur at the caecum
- 'Coffee bean' sign – inverted U-shaped bowel loops pointing towards the pelvis

PERFORATION

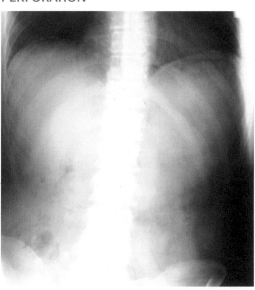

Figure 5.25 Perforated duodenal ulcer with air under the diaphragm

Features:

- Air present under one (or both) hemidiaphragm on erect chest radiograph/abdominal X-ray
- Common causes: perforated gastric or duodenal ulcer, Crohn's disease, perforated diverticulum or appendix abscess

RENAL CALCULI

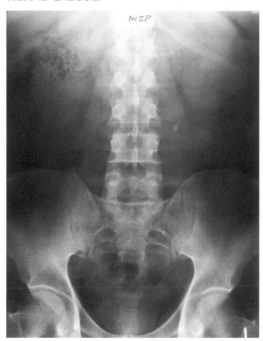

Figure 5.26 The opacity at the tip of the left transverse process of L3/4 is a ureteric calculus

Features:

- Up to 80 per cent of renal stones are radio-opaque (most common type – calcium oxalate stones)
- Uric acid stones are radiolucent
- Abdominal X-ray centred on kidney, ureters and bladder is called KUB film and may be performed with contrast to assess for renal tract obstruction (intravenous urogram)
- Stones often seen in renal calyces but small stones may pass down ureters

GALL BLADDER

- Gallstones can sometimes be seen on the plain abdominal film
- If gas-forming organisms are present within the biliary tree causing emphysematous cholecystitis, the air can be seen filling the bile ducts

URINALYSIS

A urine dipstick is a cheap, quick and simple way of testing for infections of the urinary tract as well as helping diagnose renal, urological and metabolic diseases.

SPECIFIC GRAVITY

- Essentially detects how concentrated the urine is
- Normal range: 1.010 to 1.030
- High specific gravity is caused by dehydration, ketoacidosis or proteinuria
- Low specific gravity is caused by diabetes insipidus, renal failure and pyelonephritis

pH

- Normal range: 4.8 to 7.5
- Very acidic urine may be due to diabetic ketoacidosis, diarrhoea and starvation
- Very alkaline urine may be due to urinary tract infection (UTI), vomiting and rarely renal tubular acidosis.

HAEMATURIA

This may be macroscopic (blood-stained urine) or microscopic (urine looks normal – red blood cells on microscopy).

Causes include:

- Renal disease – glomerulonephritis
- Infection – UTI, pyelonephritis
- Malignancy – bladder, renal carcinoma
- Obstruction – urolithiasis
- False positives – menstruation, myoglobinuria

Note:

- In the presence of other indicators of infection (leucocytes, nitrites or clinical symptoms) the mid-stream urine sample should be sent for microscopy and culture
- Persistent haematuria in patients under 45 years of age should be referred to a nephrologist or to a urologist if the patient is over 45

PROTEINURIA

- Urine dipstick can detect as little as 30 mg/dL of protein.
- Causes of leakage of protein into the urine include:
  - Renovascular disease
  - Glomerular disease, e.g. glomerulonephritis, diabetes, systemic lupus erythematosus
  - Tubular renal disease, e.g. hypertension, non-steroidal anti-inflammatory drugs (NSAIDs)

Note:

- The urine should be sent for total protein-creatinine ratio (TPCR) and microscopy and culture
- Proteinuria > TPCR 100 mg/mmol, or proteinuria > TPCR 45 mg/mmol with microscopic haematuria, should be referred for further investigation

GLYCOSURIA

Glucose should be undetectable in the urine and its presence is a good screening tool for diabetes mellitus

- Glycosuria is not diagnostic of diabetes
- Renal glycosuria, can lead to sugar within the urine but normal glucose levels in the plasma
- Venous blood glucose levels should be checked and HbA_{1c} if appropriate

KETONURIA

The presence of ketones in the urine suggests the breakdown of fat, in place of carbohydrate, as the major source of energy.

Ketonuria is detectable in:

- Pregnancy
- Starvation
- The acutely unwell patient (stress response)
- Diabetes (where ketoacidosis would be a concern)

NITRITES

Nitrites are produced by the breakdown of urinary nitrates by bacteria – usually Gram-negative species.

Note:

- Not a very sensitive test for infection: patients with symptoms of infection should have microscopy performed even if dipstick is negative for nitrites
- A positive test, in correlation with clinical suspicion, warrants treatment for UTI
- False positives occur when strips are exposed to the air for a prolonged period or if the patient is on vitamin C supplementation

LEUCOCYTES

- Urinary dipsticks detect leucocyte-esterase produced by neutrophils, suggesting pyuria
- It is slightly more sensitive, but less specific, than testing for nitrites
- Correlation with clinical symptoms is necessary, and microscopy and culture are required
- Positive leucocytes and positive culture – urinary tract infection or contaminant
- Positive leucocytes and negative culture, e.g. bladder cancer, renal stones, tuberculosis

ARTERIAL BLOOD GASES

Arterial blood gas (ABG) sampling is a vital tool in assessing the acid–base balance of critically ill patients as well as measuring the adequacy of respiration.

NORMAL VALUES

Table 5.2 Normal values of arterial blood gases

pH	7.35–7.45
pCO_2	4.5–6.0 kPa
pO_2	10–14 kPa (room air)
HCO_3^-	22–26 mmol/L
Base excess	+3 to −3 mmol/L
SaO_2	>95 per cent
Na^+	135–146 mmol/L
K^+	3.5–5.1 mmol/L
Cl^-	95–105 mmol/L
Ca^{2+} (ionized)	1.0–1.2 mmol/L
Haemoglobin	11.5–15 g/dL (female) 13–16 g/dL (male)

Note: values may vary slightly depending on equipment used.

INTERPRETING ABNORMAL RESULTS

pH

- pH <7.35 – the patient is acidotic
- pH >7.45 – the patient is alkalotic
- pH between 7.35 and 7.45 is normal, but there may have been an acid–base disturbance which has been *compensated* for by other mechanisms.

Carbon Dioxide (CO_2)

- This is determined by ventilation
- If the CO_2 is high (>6 kPa) there is under-ventilation of the lungs and any coexisting acidosis is termed 'respiratory'
- If the CO_2 is low (<4.5 Pa) there is over-ventilation (and any concurrent acidosis would therefore be 'metabolic' in origin)
- Over-ventilation may occur to compensate a metabolic acidosis by increasing CO_2 removal

Bicarbonate (HCO_3^-)

- This gives an indication of the metabolic component of the acid–base balance.
- A low standard bicarbonate (<22 mmol/L) indicates a metabolic acidosis.
- A high standard bicarbonate shows either a metabolic alkalosis or an attempt by the kidneys to correct a chronic respiratory acidosis.

Oxygen (O_2)

- Consider the partial pressure of oxygen in relation to the amount of inspired oxygen
- While a PaO_2 on room air FiO_2 0.21 should be 10–14 kPa, the same results would indicate inadequate ventilation with a corresponding inspired oxygen concentration of 100 per cent, for example.

ANION GAP

- The anion gap represents the difference between the cations (positively charged particles) and the anions (negatively charged particles):
  - Anion gap = $([Na^+] + [K^+]) - ([Cl^-] + [HCO_3^-])$

- Normally this should be 8–16 mmol/L.
- This calculates an artificial value of the unmeasured ions in the plasma and can be helpful in determining the cause of a metabolic acidosis – see Table 5.4

Table 5.3 Common patterns on arterial blood gases

	pH	$PaCO_2$	HCO_3^-
Respiratory acidosis	↓	↑	Normal or ↑
Respiratory alkalosis	↑	↓	Normal or ↓
Metabolic acidosis	↓	Normal or ↓	↓
Metabolic alkalosis	↑	Normal	↑

Table 5.4 Causes of abnormal arterial blood gases

Common causes of respiratory acidosis (due to alveolar hypoventilation)

Respiratory failure	Chronic obstructive pulmonary disease
	Asthma
	Obesity hypoventilation
Neuromuscular	Motor neurone disease
	Guillain–Barré syndrome
	Amyotrophic lateral sclerosis
	Myasthenia gravis
Drugs	Opiates
	Sedatives
	Muscle relaxants

Common causes of respiratory alkalosis (due to alveolar hyperventilation)

Psychogenic	Hyperventilation (anxiety, stress)
Drugs	Salicylate overdose
Metabolic	Acute liver failure
Respiratory	Pulmonary embolus
	Pneumonia
	Asthma
Central nervous system	Stroke
	Haemorrhage

Common causes of metabolic acidosis (due to acid gain or alkali loss)

Common causes with an *increased* anion gap

Metabolic	Diabetic ketoacidosis
	Lactic acidosis (sepsis, tissue hypoperfusion)
	Renal failure
Drugs	Salicylate overdose
	Methanol poisoning
	Ethylene glycol poisoning
	Metformin

Common causes with a *normal* anion gap

Gastrointestinal	Diarrhoea
	Large losses via stoma or fistula
Metabolic	Renal tubular acidosis

Common causes of metabolic alkalosis (due to acid loss or alkali gain)

Gastrointestinal	Vomiting
Metabolic	Hypokalaemia
Drugs	Alkali ingestion

SERUM ELECTROLYTES

This daily task for a junior doctor can provide vital keys to the diagnosis and the progression of an illness.

NORMAL RANGES

(**Note:** these vary slightly between hospitals)

Table 5.5 Normal ranges

Sodium (Na$^+$)	135–145 mmol/L
Potassium (K$^+$)	3.5–5 mmol/ L
Magnesium (Mg^{2+})	0.7–1.00 mmol/L
Chloride (Cl$^-$)	96–106 mmol/L
Bicarbonate (HCO$_3{}^-$)	22–32 mmol/L
Corrected calcium (Ca^{2+})	2.20–2.60 mmol/L
Phosphate (PO$_4{}^{3-}$)	0.8–1.4 mmol/L

HYPONATRAEMIA

Symptoms

- Often asymptomatic
- Nausea/vomiting
- Headache
- Confusion or agitation
- Seizures
- Coma

Causes

(Mild hyponatraemia >125 mmol/L, severe hyponatraemia <125 mmol/L)

- Pseudohyponatraemia
    - Hyperlipidaemia
    - Hyperproteinaemia (e.g. myeloma)
- True hyponatraemia (classified by fluid status):
    - Hypovolaemia
        - Vomiting, diarrhoea, burns
        - Diuretics
        - Hypoadrenalism
        - Salt losing nephropathy
    - Euvolaemia
        - Syndrome of inappropriate antidiuretic hormone secretion (SIADH)*
        - Hypothyroidism
    - Hypervolaemia
        - Congestive cardiac failure
        - Cirrhotic liver disease
        - Nephrotic syndrome

*There are multiple causes of SIADH including:

- Respiratory disease (pneumonia, tuberculosis),
- Malignancy (bronchial, pancreatic, duodenal)
- Intracerebral (tumours, abscesses, haemorrhage, inflammatory CNS disorders, trauma, surgery, fits, encephalitis)
- Drugs (phenothiazines, tricyclics, serotonin selective reuptake inhibitors)

SIADH is a **diagnosis of exclusion**. The following criteria must be met:

- Euvolaemic hyponatraemia
- Not on diuretics
- Urine Na >20 mmol/L
- Normal thyroid and adrenal function
- Normal cardiac, hepatic and renal function
- Inappropriately concentrated urine (urine osmolality > plasma osmolality)

HYPERNATRAEMIA

Symptoms

- Thirst
- Lethargy and malaise
- Confusion
- Seizures
- Coma

Causes

- Dehydration (vomiting, burns, diarrhoea, diuretics)
- Excess saline (iatrogenic)
- Cushing's syndrome
- Diabetes insipidus (if patient cannot maintain fluid intake)
  - Central
  - Nephrogenic

HYPOKALAEMIA

Symptoms

- Muscle weakness and cramps
- Paraesthesia
- Palpitations (caused by cardiac arrhythmias)
- Cardiac arrest

Causes

- Medication – diuretics, laxatives, steroids, insulin
- Vomiting
- Diarrhoea
- Parenteral nutrition or refeeding syndrome
- Rare causes: Conn's syndrome (hyperaldosteronism), Bartter's syndrome

HYPERKALAEMIA

Symptoms

- Often asymptomatic
- Occasionally muscle cramps or muscle paralysis including respiratory paralysis
- Cardiac arrhythmias/arrest

Causes

- Pseudohyperkalaemia:
  - Haemolysed blood sample
  - Old blood sample
  - Thrombocytosis or leucocytosis
- True hyperkalaemia:
  - Medication – potassium-sparing diuretics (e.g. spironolactone), angiotensin-converting enzyme inhibitors
  - Excess potassium replacement (iatrogenic)
  - Renal failure
  - Acidosis
  - Rhabdomyolysis
  - Addison's disease (primary hypoadrenalism)

HYPOCALCAEMIA

Symptoms

- Tingling and numbness
- Tetany
- Cardiac arrhythmias, ischaemia, failure
- Bronchospasm, dyspnoea

Causes

- Hypoalbuminaemia
- Vitamin D deficiency
- Hypoparathyroidism
- Drugs, e.g. fluoride, proton pump inhibitors
- Pancreatitis
- Renal disease
- Massive blood transfusion

HYPERCALCAEMIA

Symptoms

'Bones, stones, abdominal moans and psychic groans'

- Muscle/joint aches and pain
- Urinary calculi
- Abdominal pain, constipation, vomiting
- Cardiac arrhythmias
- Depression

Causes

- Hyperparathyroidism
- Malignancy
- Sarcoidosis
- Drugs, e.g. thiazides, lithium

URAEMIA/HIGH UREA

Symptoms

- Fatigue
- Pruritus
- Anorexia
- Confusion
- Muscle weakness
- Pericarditis
- Encephalopathy
- Gastrointestinal bleeding

Causes

- Renal failure (with concomitant raised creatinine):
  - Acute
  - Chronic

CEREBROSPINAL FLUID

INDICATIONS FOR CEREBROSPINAL FLUID (CSF) SAMPLING

To aid the diagnosis of:

- Meningitis (bacterial, viral, tuberculosis)
- Subarachnoid haemorrhage
- Multiple sclerosis
- Guillain–Barré syndrome
- Malignancy

COMMON PATTERNS

Meningitis

- Not all the criteria in Table 5.6 need to be met to make a diagnosis

Table 5.6 Criteria for meningitis

	Normal	Bacterial	Viral	Tuberculosis
Appearance	Crystal clear	Cloudy, turbid	Clear	Yellow
Neutrophils	0	100–10 000	<100	Variable
Lymphocytes	0	<100	10–10 000	Increased
CSF: plasma glucose ratio	66 per cent	<40 per cent	Normal	Low
Protein	0.15–0.40g/L	>1 g/L	0.4–1 g/l	Increased
Culture	Negative	Positive	Negative	Acid fast bacilli

Subarachnoid haemorrhage

- Straw-coloured, pink or blood-tinged fluid
- Consistently high red cell count in sequential bottles (by contrast, the red cell count will fall sequentially in a traumatic tap)
- Positive xanthochromia (red blood cell decomposition products, including bilirubin)

Multiple sclerosis

- High CSF protein
- Oligoclonal bands on electrophoresis

Guillain–Barré

- High CSF protein (rising in sequential samples)
- <10 mononuclear cells

Malignancy (lepto-meningeal disease)

- High protein and cell count
- Malignant cells

PLEURAL FLUID

Pleural fluid sampling (thoracentesis) is essential in narrowing the large number of causes of an effusion.

EXUDATES AND TRANSUDATES

- An exudate is classified as pleural fluid with protein >30 g/L
- A transudate is defined as pleural fluid with <30 g/L of protein
- In borderline cases Light's criteria are used – these define an exudate by one or more of the following criteria:
  - Pleural fluid total protein:serum total protein ratio >0.5
  - Pleural fluid lactate dehydrogenase (LDH):serum LDH ratio >0.6
  - Pleural fluid LDH >66 per cent (two thirds) of the upper limit of normal of the serum LDH

Table 5.7 Causes of exudative and transudative pleural effusions

Exudate	Transudate
Malignancy (see 'Cytology' below)	Cardiac failure (most common)
Pneumonia	Hypoproteinaemia:
Empyema	Liver cirrhosis
Tuberculosis	Nephrotic syndrome
Pulmonary embolism	Hypothyroidism
Connective tissue disorders:	Peritoneal dialysis
Rheumatoid arthritis	Rare:
Systemic lupus erythematosus	Meigs' syndrome
Systemic sclerosis	Constrictive pericarditis
Rare:	Pulmonary embolism
Pancreatitis	
Drug-induced effusions	
Yellow nail syndrome	

LOW pH AND GLUCOSE

The causes of pleural effusions with a low pH (<7.2) and low glucose (<3.3 mmol/L) are:

- Infection – complicated parapneumonic effusions or empyema
- Malignancy
- Connective tissue diseases
- Tuberculosis

AMYLASE

An amylase-rich effusion is most likely to indicate acute pancreatitis or rupture of the oesophagus.

CYTOLOGY

Malignant cells may be due to:

- Bronchial carcinoma
- Breast cancer
- Ovarian cancer
- Haematological malignancies
- Gastrointestinal tract tumour
- Mesothelioma

OTHER CAUSES OF PLEURAL EFFUSION

- Chylothorax: due to accumulation of lymphatic fluid in the chest cavity:
  - This is usually caused by leakage or blockage of the thoracic duct
  - Surgery, trauma or lymphoma are the main causes
  - Typically the pleural fluid triglyceride and cholesterol levels are very high
- Haemothorax:
  - Collection of blood in the pleural space is usually as a consequence of trauma
  - Rare but potentially fatal

PULMONARY FUNCTION TESTS

Pulmonary function tests (PFTs) are a set of breathing tests, usually including spirometry, which are used to measure the volume and function of the lungs.

They can be helpful in:

- Diagnosing respiratory conditions
- Predicting prognosis according to severity
- Assessing the effects of bronchodilators

PEAK FLOW EXPIRATORY RATE

- The peak flow device is a hand-held, portable device (mini-Wright peak flow) which measures the maximum flow rate achieved during a forced expiration

- Peak expiratory flow rate (PEFR) is measured in litres per minute. The best recorded measurement after three attempts is compared to a nomogram which takes into account the patient's age, sex and height (see Figure 5.27).

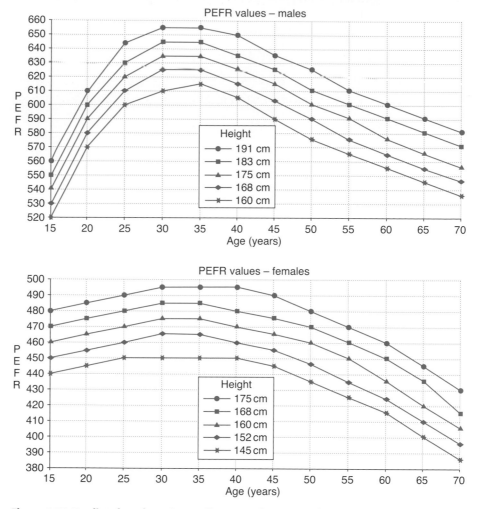

Figure 5.27 Predicted peak expiratory flow rates for men and women (redrawn with permission from gp-training.net [www.gp-training.net])

- PEFR monitoring is a very useful bedside test. It can assess:
  - The severity of an acute asthma attack
  - Diurnal patterns
  - Responsiveness to treatment

SPIROMETRY

- This is the most common formal PFT
- It involves breathing in and out of a mouthpiece attached to a sensor
- It measures the volume of air forced out by maximal expiration after taking a maximal inspiration and is displayed as a plot of volume (litres) against time (seconds)
- The volume, measured in litres, is the forced vital capacity (FVC)

- The volume expired within the first second of this forced manoeuvre is defined as the forced expiratory volume in 1 second (FEV$_1$)
- An increase in the FEV$_1$ of more than 12 per cent (or 200 mL) after administration of a bronchodilator is considered to show significant reversibility.

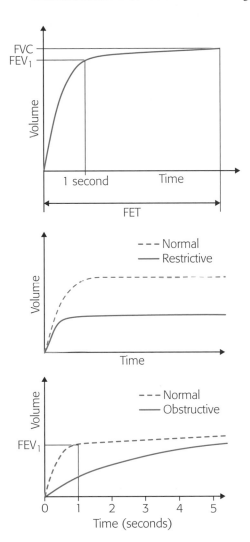

Figure 5.28 Normal FEV$_1$ to FVC ratio should be 75–80 per cent in adults

Figure 5.29 In this illustration the FEV$_1$ is lowered but in proportion to the reduced FVC, maintaining the FEV$_1$:FVC ratio

Figure 5.30 Although both the FEV$_1$ and the FVC are reduced, the FEV$_1$ is relatively more reduced, leading to a reduction in the FEV$_1$:FVC ratio to less than 80 per cent

Table 5.8 Changes in obstructive and restrictive lung disease

	Obstructive defect	Restrictive defect
Forced expiratory volume in 1 second (FEV1)	Decreased	Variable
Forced vital capacity (FVC)	Decreased (or normal)	Decreased
FEV1:FVC	Decreased (<80 per cent)	Normal or increased
Total lung capacity	Normal or increased	Decreased
Residual volume	Normal or increased	Decreased

FLOW–VOLUME LOOPS

- Flow–volume loops display maximal inspiratory flow and maximal expiratory flow against time
- The shape of the loop can be characteristic of certain disease patterns

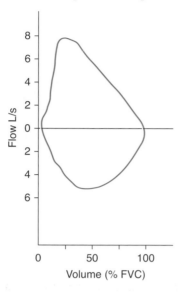

Figure 5.31 Normal flow–volume loop (redrawn with permission from AnaesthesiaUK [www.frca.co.uk])

Normal

- Expiration is shown above the line
- Inspiration is shown below the line
- FVC, PEFR, total lung capacity and residual volume can all be calculated

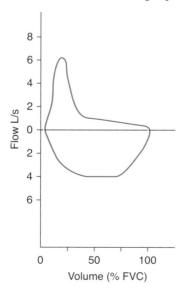

Figure 5.32 Flow–volume loop in chronic obstructive pulmonary disease (redrawn with permission from AnaesthesiaUK [www.frca.co.uk])

Chronic Obstructive Pulmonary Disease

- Classically there is a concave shape to the expiratory loop after maximal expiration demonstrating the difficulty of forcing breath out with airways collapse
- The inspiratory loop is often a normal shape but of a reduced size

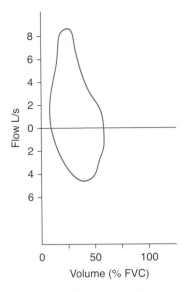

Figure 5.33 Flow–volume loop in restrictive lung defect (redrawn with permission from AnaesthesiaUK [www.frca.co.uk])

Restrictive Disease

- The lung volumes are smaller so the loop is much narrower but the shape is usually preserved

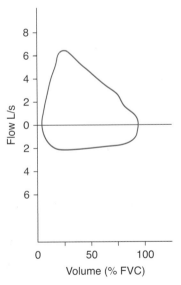

Figure 5.34 Flow–volume loop in fixed upper airways obstruction (redrawn with permission from AnaesthesiaUK [www.frca.co.uk])

Upper Airway Obstruction

- Flow is limited in both inspiratory and expiratory phases often with a plateau phase, creating a more rectangular shape

Communication skills

CT/MRI SCAN

Cross-sectional imaging is commonly performed on both outpatients and inpatients. Being asked to explain the procedure is a common request in finals.

INTRODUCTION

- Introduce yourself by name and position
- Confirm the patient's name
- Ensure they are sitting comfortably, alongside and not behind a desk
- Ask what they understand having a scan involves
- Try to elicit any ideas/concerns/expectations ('ICE')

EXPLAINING REASONS FOR THE TEST

- Explain the indication for the test in lay language, e.g. 'We want to find out why you're coughing up the blood'
- Try to give a list of the diagnoses that may result from the test. Even if suspecting malignancy, mention this to the patient, so that if this is confirmed, it is not a complete surprise.

EXPLAINING THE TEST ITSELF

- The aim of the test is to create pictures of the inside of the patient by using a scanner
- It involves lying on a flat bed and then moving into the machine
- A drip may be placed into the arm to allow a special dye to be given to make the pictures clearer
- The whole procedure takes up to 20 minutes for a computed tomography (CT) scan and up to about 45 minutes for magnetic resonance imaging (MRI), depending on the complexity of the scan
- A CT scanner uses radiation to produce the pictures, whereas an MRI scanner uses a powerful magnet
- MRI scanners may make loud noises, so earplugs may be provided

CAUTIONS

- MRI:
  - The tunnel is closed and so may produce problems for those with claustrophobia
  - The powerful magnet may interfere with pacemakers or internal defibrillators – ask if the patient has one
  - Joint prostheses – unless recently inserted – pose no problems
  - Metal foreign bodies, such as shrapnel or metal fragments within the eye, can cause problems if they move when exposed to the strong magnetic field
  - Chronic renal impairment may cause difficulties if any intravenous contrast is used
- CT
  - As radiation is used to produce the images, there is a probable small additional risk of malignancy
  - If there is any chance the patient could be pregnant, she must have a pregnancy test before the procedure
  - Intravenous contrast can lead to a decrease in renal function – this is more pronounced if the patient has known chronic renal impairment and/or diabetes mellitus.

FOLLOW UP

- A radiologist will look at the images after the scan is complete and produce a report which will go to the patient's referring doctor
- Any questions about the results should be directed at the person who requested the scan

FURTHER INFORMATION

- Offer an information leaflet if one is available
- Ask if the patient has any questions

ENDOSCOPY

Visualization of the gastrointestinal tract or respiratory tree with an endoscope is a common procedure, performed in most hospitals. Remember, although you should be able to explain the nature of these procedures, you should not obtain formal consent for them, as this will be done by the endoscopist/bronchoscopist.

INTRODUCTION

- Introduce yourself by name and position
- Confirm the patient's name
- Ensure they are sitting comfortably, alongside and not behind a desk
- Find out what the patient knows about the suggested procedure
- Try to elicit any ideas/concerns/expectations ('ICE')

INFORMATION GIVING

You should explain:

- The purpose of the examination, e.g. 'We want to look at the lining of the gullet and stomach to see why you've been vomiting blood'

- The endoscope is about the size of the patient's little finger and has a camera and small light within it
- The procedure is performed under sedation or local anaesthesia (topical lidocaine spray) as per patient preference. Some patients do not remember having the procedure at all as an effect of the sedation
- The aim of sedation is not to render the patient unconscious, just to relax the patient
- The procedure usually takes about 10 minutes
- Some samples may be taken during the procedure – these do not hurt and allow a doctor to look at the material under a microscope

COMPLICATIONS

- Very safe procedures
- Common side effects of gastroscopy are sore throat and bloating (due to the air introduced during the procedure)
- Explain that it is usual to cough during a bronchoscopy as the lungs are being irritated
- Rare side effects include drug reactions, bleeding or very occasionally perforation
- Explain the implications of these, i.e. 'In the unlikely event we do make a hole in the stomach, gullet or windpipe, you would need to stay in hospital and may even need an operation'

RESULTS

- Some results will be available immediately after the procedure when the effects of any sedation have worn off. The doctor will be able to say what he or she has seen with the naked eye
- Any findings may need confirmation with histological examination, which usually takes about a week
- The patient should contact the doctor who requested the test for the final results

ANY QUESTIONS/CONCERNS?

Allow the patient an opportunity to voice any concerns or questions they might have.

PERCUTANEOUS CORONARY INTERVENTION

Therapies applied directly to the coronary arteries using catheters have revolutionized cardiology. Thousands of patients undergo percutaneous coronary intervention (PCI) every year and junior doctors are often responsible for explaining what is involved.

INTRODUCTION

- Introduce yourself by name and position
- Confirm the patient's name
- Ensure they are sitting comfortably, alongside and not behind a desk
- Find out what the patient knows about the suggested procedure
- Try to elicit any ideas/concerns/expectations ('ICE')
- Use lay language as far as possible

INFORMATION GIVING

Explain:

- The purpose of the examination, e.g. 'We want to look at the blood vessels of your heart to see why you've been having chest pain'
- The procedure is carried out by puncturing one of the arteries in the groin or the wrist, under local anaesthesia to numb the area
- A very fine tube is inserted into the artery and then fed into the arteries of the heart. Dye is then injected into the arteries and X-ray pictures taken to see if there are any narrowings
- The patient should not feel any pain inside their chest as there are no nerves inside the arteries
- Treatment options: 'If there is a narrowing we can treat we might want to stretch it out with a small balloon and then put a tiny spring inside to keep the artery open'
- It can take up to an hour, and sometimes longer, depending on the complexity of the procedure
- If the femoral artery is used, the patient will have to lie flat after the procedure until the bleeding has stopped
- For diagnostic angiography, the patient can go home that day. For therapeutic intervention (stent insertion) most hospitals admit patients overnight for observation
- If a stent is placed, the patient will need to take aspirin and clopidogrel together for at least a month, and maybe up to 1 year

COMPLICATIONS

- PCI are usually very safe procedures
- Common side effects are bleeding from the puncture site and a flushing sensation as the radiological contrast is injected
- Rare side effects include drug reactions (including contrast nephropathy), pericardial effusion, or rupture of a coronary artery:
  - Explain the implications of these, i.e. 'In the unlikely event we do make a hole in the artery, you would need to stay in hospital and may well need an emergency operation'
  - Do not forget to mention the risk of gastrointestinal bleeding months later from the dual antiplatelet therapy.

RESULTS

- Results will be available immediately after the procedure. The operator should be able to tell the patient the condition of their arteries and what therapies have been carried out
- Sometimes, particularly in more complex cases, the X-rays are reviewed later on, and the results from these discussions should be available at the next clinic visit

ANY QUESTIONS/CONCERNS?

- Allow the patient an opportunity to voice any concerns or questions they might have
- Provide the patient with an information leaflet and website addresses for further reference

DIABETES

Diabetes is an increasingly prevalent illness. In type 2 diabetes mellitus if lifestyle measures alone have failed, treatment with medication is usually required. For those with type 1 diabetes, who often present for the first time very unwell, explaining treatment is an important part of a junior doctor's job.

INTRODUCTION

- Introduce yourself by name and position
- Adopt an open body posture
- Ask what the patient understands about diabetic issues such as:
  - Diet
  - Blood sugar control and monitoring
  - Complications
- Ask if they have any ideas/concerns/expectations ('ICE')

TYPE 1 DIABETES

Background

Explain:

- The pathophysiology of type 1 diabetes: that the pancreas, which secretes insulin, to control the blood sugar levels, has stopped producing insulin
- How the pancreas usually responds to a meal by releasing insulin into the blood
- As the pancreas is not working properly, the patient will need regular insulin to prevent them from becoming very unwell
- The dose of insulin can be tailored to what the patient has eaten, just as the pancreas would respond to the size of the meal
- That regular blood sugar monitoring will be needed in order to make sure that good glucose control is achieved and the reasons for this

Insulin

Explain:

- Insulin is usually stored in the fridge
- The syringes usually have a dial to allow the patient to select the amount of insulin injected
- The needles are very fine and cause very little pain
- Rotation of injection sites is advisable to avoid lipohypertrophy (accumulation of fat under the skin)
- The exact timing of injections will vary according to the preparation prescribed. Short-acting insulins are usually taken with just before food
- Sharps should be appropriately disposed of into a yellow bin (supplied by their pharmacist)

Blood sugar monitoring

Explain:

- Advise regular monitoring
- Explain how the automatic lancet works (a small needle on a spring). The side of the finger is the least painful and most accessible place for this
- A diary can often be helpful, especially when beginning treatment, to relate blood sugar levels to injected insulin doses
- Sharps should be disposed of into a yellow bin

Hypoglycaemia

Explain:

- If too much insulin is taken, explain that the patient may become agitated, drowsy or even unconscious
- The treatment for this is a sugary drink or food which can relieve symptoms quickly or glucagon in emergency situations
- The patient may want to inform family members what to do if they are found unconscious. Some patients keep intramuscular glucagon at home for use in this event

Hyperglycaemia

Explain:

- If hyperglycaemia is noted, the patient should:
  - Adjust insulin dosage
  - Monitor urine with dipsticks for ketones
  - Attend hospital if unable to control glucose levels and very unwell
- Sick days and exercise:
  - Patients should take their blood sugars more frequently when unwell as insulin requirements increase although food intake may be compromised
  - Uncontrollable hyperglycaemia may occur during illness and hospitalization may be required
  - Exercise is likely to increase the amount of insulin required for 24–48 hours. Carbohydrate and insulin dosing should be adjusted accordingly

TYPE 2 DIABETES

Background

Explain:

- The pathophysiology of type 2 diabetes: the body does not respond as well to insulin as it used to and that glucose remains in the blood, in higher than normal concentrations
- That the pancreas, which secretes insulin, to control the blood sugar levels, is not secreting enough for the body, leading to raised sugar levels
- How the pancreas usually responds to a meal by releasing insulin into the blood
- As the pancreas is not working properly, the patient will need regular tablets or insulin to help prevent the development of serious complications
- That regular blood sugar monitoring is advisable

Tablets

- The agent of choice for patients who are overweight and have normal renal function is metformin:

○   Mention that this increases the sensitivity of the cells to insulin
○   Hypoglycaemia (low blood sugar) is typically not a feature
○   Diarrhoea is a common side effect
- The other first-line agents are the sulphonylureas such as gliclazide; these can cause hypoglycaemia
- Longer-term other medication such as aspirin, blood pressure and cholesterol-lowering tablets may be beneficial in preventing complications

Insulin
See above.

Hypoglycaemia
See above.

Follow-up
- Regular follow-up with a diabetes specialist or general practitioner is recommended
- This includes blood tests, blood pressure and urinalysis
- Patients should regularly attend a podiatrist and ophthalmologist to monitor for complications

Lifestyle
- It is imperative to emphasize the importance of a healthy diet, exercise and weight loss, which will delay and even prevent the occurrence of major complications
- Smoking is strongly discouraged

Long term complications of diabetes
- Macrovascular i.e. stroke, heart attack, peripheral vascular disease
- Microvascular i.e. eye disease, renal disease and neuropathy

DIAGNOSING CANCER

Patients fear the diagnosis of cancer immensely. It has terrible connotations to many people, who often incorrectly relate it to a painful, unpleasant death. The way in which patients are told of their diagnosis can have a significant impact on their psychological well-being.

INTRODUCTION
- Introduce yourself by name and position
- Ensure the environment is private, quiet and free from interruption
- Give your bleep to another member of the team
- Ensure that a trained nurse is present to support the patient
- Use lay language as far as possible

BREAKING THE NEWS
- Enquire how much the patient knows about their current medical problems

- Ask if anything in particular is worrying them: they may broach the topic of cancer themselves
- Explain that you have some bad news for the patient to allow them a moment to prepare themselves
- Ask if they would like a relative present
- If they do not bring up cancer themselves, go on to talk about the evidence you have that the patient has a malignancy: 'I'm afraid the scan you had shows some growths on the liver. It's likely that they are cancerous'
- Do not be afraid to the use the word cancer: patients have a right to know what is wrong with them. Otherwise patients sometimes do not equate 'growths', 'shadows', or 'lumps' with cancer and can leave the consultation without understanding what you have been trying to say
- If the patient becomes distressed, pause and allow them a little time. Hand them a tissue if needed
- Remember that after you have told them about the cancer and where it is, they will take in very little of what you say for the rest of the consultation

TREATMENT

- Most patients are anxious to know what can be done about their disease
- Specific details of treatment are best discussed with an oncologist. However, it is important to mention broadly whether there are treatment options, e.g. surgery, chemotherapy, radiotherapy or whether treatment will be focused on symptoms
- Never say that there is no treatment available, even with widespread metastatic disease, as there is always some symptomatic support that can be provided
- Explain how you will organize their ongoing treatment, e.g. referring to a multidisciplinary team meeting, with a phone call to the patient afterwards or with a clinic appointment.

LIFE EXPECTANCY

- Some, but certainly not all, patients want to know how long they can expect to live. This can be crucially important information in terms of planning financial, personal and funeral arrangements
- It is very hard to predict when someone will die, unless they are at the very end of the illness
- The best strategy to deal with this is to give advice along the lines of: 'Every patient is different, but most people in your position could expect to live for several weeks/months/years. Some of course will live longer than this, but others will not be so lucky'

FEAR OF DEATH AND DYING

- Patients are often terrified that they will die, unsupported and in pain
- Reassurance about the support services available, e.g. general practitioner, Macmillan nurses, palliative care team is very helpful in allaying these fears
- Offer to have a Macmillan nurse visit them either in hospital or at home to address any issues that they may have that they cannot think of now

ANY QUESTIONS

- Ask if the patient has any questions
- Explain it is quite common to think of questions later on as the news will have been a big shock
- Ask the patient to write down any questions for you or another team member to answer later

DO NOT RESUSCITATE ORDER

The mention of a 'do not resuscitate' (DNR) order can be an emotive time for patients, relatives and medical staff. Sensitive handing of a difficult area is an important part of a hospital doctor's job.

INTRODUCTION

- Introduce yourself by name and position
- Ensure you are in a private environment where you cannot be interrupted
- Ask for a nurse to be present
- If possible, give your bleep to another member of staff

DISCUSSION

- Begin by ascertaining what the patient/relatives know about the current clinical state and what the prospects are
- Move on to begin explaining the purpose of cardiopulmonary resuscitation (CPR)
- Explain that if the heart or lungs were to stop working due to underlying illness, the medical team feel that it might not be appropriate to perform CPR as a meaningful recovery from such a condition is very unlikely
- Explain the disadvantages of CPR:
  - Many patients do not survive
  - Many who do survive are left in a worse clinical state than before the event
  - Very few return to their baseline function
  - It is an undignified death with many people causing a commotion around the bedside, performing invasive tests that will have no effect on the ultimate outcome
  - Television dramas, which many people relate to, bear little relation to real cardiac arrest situations, and have far higher success rates
- Make sure that the patient/relatives understand that a DNR order is not the same as withdrawing all treatment
- Clarify that it may well be appropriate to treat the patient very aggressively – but if the treatment fails, any attempt at resuscitation is likely to be futile
- Some patients themselves ask for a DNR order. These patients should be fully informed of the consequences of their decision
- It is crucial that relatives do not feel that the decision is up to them – it is a medical decision about which you are seeking their views
- Ideally everyone involved should establish a consensus about what is in the best interests of the patient

- If you cannot reach agreement with the patient or family, involve a more senior member of staff
- Ultimately the final decision lies with the medical staff and moribund patients will not be resuscitated on the request of relatives alone

COMMUNICATION WITH OTHER STAFF

- Hospitals have dedicated paperwork for DNR orders. They are usually red or pink and should be completed and filed in the front of the notes
- Inform the nurses of the decision made so that inappropriate cardiac arrest calls are avoided
- A consultant, or if unavailable a registrar, should sign DNR forms due to the implications of the order
- However, other more junior staff should feel free to have discussions with patients and their families about these issues

BREAKING BAD NEWS: DEATH OF A RELATIVE

Telling relatives about the death of a loved one is never easy, and never becomes routine like some other parts of medicine. The way in which it is done is profoundly important and makes a real difference to relatives' experience of what is always a difficult time.

INTRODUCTION

- Introduce yourself by name and position
- Ensure you are in a private environment where you cannot be interrupted
- If possible, give your bleep to another member of staff
- Ask for a member of the nursing staff to be present

DISCUSSION

- Start by signposting that you are going to deliver some bad news: 'I'm afraid I have some bad news for you'
  - ○ This allows people even a small amount of time to prepare for what is about to come
  - ○ In many instances, relatives guess by your demeanour and the tone of the conversation
- Ask them what they already know about their relative's admission to hospital
- Confirm or inform them of the sequence of events around the death
- Break the news, without using euphemisms, expressing sorrow for their loss, e.g. 'I'm sorry to tell you that your mother has died'
- Allow a moment for the news to sink in. Offer a tissue if needed
- Explain the circumstances of the death: 'She died peacefully last night and was not in any pain'
- Answer any questions that they may have
- Offer to return later if they have any further queries
- Ask whether they are content with the care that their relative received and if there are any issues surrounding the death they would like addressed. Offer to take these up with the relevant people

ADMINISTRATIVE ISSUES

- Ask the family to leave a contact number with the nurses. Explain that the bereavement office will be in contact the next working day to help arrange the paperwork
- Explain that a death certificate will be filled out which the family can take to the local Registrar in Births, Deaths and Marriages in order to register the death officially
- Ask if they would like a cremation or burial, as additional paperwork is needed
- If you are not sure of the cause of death, explain that you will have to discuss the case with the coroner (see p. 249) who might want a post-mortem. This is good practice as otherwise the request for a post-mortem can be a real shock

FINALLY

- Ask again if there are any other questions
- Provide your contact details in case further questions arise

DEATH CERTIFICATION

Source: Adapted from *Guidance for Doctors Certifying Cause of Death* (Office for National Statistics Death Certification Advisory Group, London, April 2005)

The death certificate is a legal document and knowing how to correctly complete a death certificate is a very important responsibility of a junior doctor.

CONFIRMING A DEATH

- This may be performed by doctor, or trained nurse, if the death occurred out of hours:
  - Pupils: fixed and dilated
  - Painful stimuli: no response
  - Pulse: absent carotid pulse and heart sounds (listen for 2 minutes)
  - Breathing: absent breath sounds (listen for 2 minutes)
- Document the above in the notes along with the date and the time you examined and confirmed the death
- 'Rest in peace' is often written after this

COMPLETING THE DEATH CERTIFICATE

- Only a doctor who cared for the patient during the last illness and has seen the patient within the 14 days prior to death may complete a death certificate
- All the relevant medical records should be available for filling out the form

INFORMATION REQUIRED ON THE DEATH CERTIFICATE

- Name of patient
- Date of death
- Age of patient
- Place patient died
- Date last seen by the doctor completing the certificate

You must then circle one of the following statements:

(a) The certified cause of death takes account of information obtained from post-mortem
(b) Information from post-mortem may be available later
(c) Post-mortem not being held
(d) I have reported this death to the Coroner for further action

In the majority of cases part (c) will be appropriate, unless the death has been reported to the coroner. A second statement must then be circled:

(a) Seen after death by me
(b) Seen after death by another medical practitioner but not by me
(c) Not seen after death by a medical practitioner

Cause of death

- It is good practice to discuss what will be put on the certificate as the cause of death with a senior colleague (usually consultant or registrar)
- If the cause is not known or unclear it should be discussed with the coroner (see below)
- Cause of death consists of three sections:
  - Parts 1(a), (b) and (c) relate to the immediate condition(s), which led to death
  - Part 2 relates to any important co-morbidity which may have played a part in the patient's death
- The cause of death should be as specific as possible. An example might be:
  - Part 1 (a) Bronchopneumonia
  - Part 1 (b) Chronic obstructive pulmonary disease
  - Part 2 Coronary heart disease

Note

The following are examples of modes of dying and **not** causes of death and should be avoided:

- Cardiac arrest
- Coma
- Heart failure
- Liver/renal failure
- Respiratory arrest

Do not use abbreviations – this may mean that the certificate will not be accepted by the registrar.

Industrial disease

There is a box where it should be indicated if the disease was related to employment or industrial disease, e.g. mesothelioma. This will affect compensation and pensions, and must also be reported to the coroner.

Other information

Other information required to finish the document includes:

- Your signature and surname in block capitals
- Your medical qualification

- Your address (usually the hospital)
- The date the form was filled in
- The consultant responsible for the care of the patient

REPORTING DEATHS TO THE CORONER

Certain categories of deaths must be reported to the coroner before the certificate for registration can be issued. The full list of these is located at the front of the medical certificate forms book, for reference.

- The cause of death was unknown
- The deceased was not seen by the certifying doctor *either* after death *or* within the 14 days before death
- The death was violent or unnatural or was suspicious
- The death may be due to an accident
- The death may be due to self-neglect or neglect by others
- The death may be due to an industrial disease or related to the deceased's employment
- The death may be due to an abortion
- The death occurred during an operation or before recovery from the effects of an anaesthetic
- The death may be a suicide
- The death occurred during or shortly after detention in police custody or prison

The coroner will need to know as much information relating to the case from you as possible to be able to decide if further investigation (post-mortem or inquest) is necessary:

- If the coroner is satisfied that the cause of death can be established without a post-mortem they will ask you to complete the certificate in the usual way
- If you have reported a case to the coroner, make sure you circle option 4 and initial Box A on the back of the form
- Rarely, a coroner's inquest will be necessary to allow further exploration of the cause and circumstances surrounding the death
- As one of the doctors attending to the deceased you may be required to appear at the coroner's court to give evidence or to submit a written statement

RESPONDING TO AN UNSATISFIED PATIENT

Complaints will affect most doctors at some point in their careers. Dealing with dissatisfied patients is an important skill, because if concerns can be dealt with promptly, a good doctor–patient relationship can be maintained.

INTRODUCTION
- Introduce yourself by name and position
- Ensure you are in a private environment where you cannot be interrupted
- If possible, give your bleep to another member of staff
- Ask for a member of the nursing staff to be present
- Keep your composure regardless of what is said. Do not raise your voice even if the other party becomes irate

FINDING OUT THE REASON FOR THE COMPLAINT

- Always start with an open question about what you can do to help: This is often all that is needed for the concerns about care to be expressed
- Allow the person to talk uninterrupted to express their views fully. Look attentive
- If there is criticism of you, your team, or the hospital, do not allow this to affect your personal feelings or be drawn into an argument
- Ask relevant questions so as to be absolutely clear what the issues are

RESPONDING TO A COMPLAINT

- Address each of the problems in turn in a systematic manner
- If you or the hospital has made a mistake, say sorry immediately and with conviction. This is often enough to placate even irate patients and relatives and can defuse tension
- If there are queries about items that are outside your remit, e.g. food, cleanliness, offer to pass your concerns along. Alternatively, offer to arrange a meeting with those responsible for those areas
- Do not blame individual members of staff as the facts are often not completely clear
- Mention that the Patient Advice and Liaison Service (PALS) office can help tackle any problems, and can avoid formal complaints being made
- Explain the process for making a complaint (usually in writing to the chief executive); offer to provide a leaflet to facilitate this process if required
- Confirm that even if a complaint is made, the clinical care of the patient will not be affected

FURTHER ACTIONS

- If there has been a clinical error or a serious incident, make sure you explain that you will be filling in the appropriate paperwork to ensure that the mistake is recognized
- Explaining how the same problem will not occur in future is useful both to the hospital and the patient, as many patients who have been badly treated just want to be sure the same thing does not happen to someone else
- Document the conversation and any agreed actions in the clinical notes, with a record of who was present during the meeting
- Inform your seniors/consultant of the meeting and the outcome

KEEPING PATIENT CONFIDENTIALITY

Confidentiality is paramount in maintaining the doctor–patient relationship. However, although not an absolute, doctors should think very carefully before breaking this covenant. A common difficult scenario occurs when patients' relatives want to know clinical information without the consent of the patient.

INTRODUCTION

- Introduce yourself and ask family members to do the same
- Arrange a quiet meeting room where you will not be interrupted
- Keep calm, no matter what is said, and remain polite throughout

DISCUSSION

- Ask what the family would like to know
- Find out what they know already
- Remember, if the patient is competent, you cannot disclose any information about their treatment without the consent of the patient
- The best way to overcome this obstacle is to ask the patient if they mind you discussing their condition with the family
  - If they object, then politely decline any requests for information, saying that the patient should be able to explain directly to them and that you are not allowed to discuss confidential matters with them
- It is not uncommon for doctors to be asked to keep information secret from patients, particularly when the diagnosis is serious, e.g. cancer
  - This is unethical if the patient is competent – every person has the right to know about their own state of health
  - An approach saying that you can involve the family when breaking any bad news, if the patient consents, often provides a satisfactory compromise
- In the case of an incompetent patient, you are often obliged to break confidentiality to act in the best interests of the patient by discussing their care with interested parties such as the family or carers

BREAKING CONFIDENTIALITY

- This is always a difficult area. If you feel that other people are at a serious threat from information divulged during a consultation, then you are at liberty to pass this information on. For example, if a patient says that they are going to commit a serious crime, then you are obliged to report this to the police for further action
- Breaking confidentiality should be regarded as a last resort. It is often helpful to have advice from your defence union when dealing with 'grey area' cases

FOLLOW-UP

- Offer the relatives and patient a chance to meet the consultant responsible for their care if they have further questions or concerns
- Provide them with the contact details for the PALS office for further advice

EXPLAINING STATISTICS TO PATIENTS

Quantifying risk is found difficult even by highly educated people. Many would not go skydiving owing to fear of death but would not think twice about driving their car, which is arguably more dangerous.

Much of modern medicine is now based on risks and chances: it is important to inform patients as much as possible of these when discussing difficult decisions.

INTRODUCTION

- Introduce yourself by name and position
- Adopt an open body posture
- Use lay language as far as possible

INFORMATION GIVING

- Risk is a difficult concept. Each person weighs a perceived risk in a different way
- There are many situations in which patients need to know information about risk in order to make an informed decision about a procedure or treatment
- A 1 in 2000 perforation risk at colonoscopy may seem remote to most people. However, this may seem unacceptable to someone who is terrified of a subsequent operation
- Your job is to explain a risk in a manner in which the patient can understand. It is often helpful to relate this to events that the patient can relate to

---

BOX 6.1 COMMON STATISTICS

Event	Chance
Winning National Lottery	1 in 14 000 000 (approximate)
Being struck by lightning	1 in 3 000 000 (approximate)
Odds of guessing a four-digit padlock code	1 in 10 000
A child having the same birthday as their parent	1 in 365
Choosing the right number in a game of roulette	1 in 37
Dying of a heart attack	1 in 5
Tossing a coin (heads or tails)	1 in 2

- The personal difference between a 1 in 10 000 risk and 1 in 50 000 risk is impossible to gauge. Apart from using analogies, simplifying matters into those that are rare and those that are common is often helpful to patients
- Remember that those risks that may seem rare and unimportant to you may be crucially important to the patient, e.g. a concert pianist may not wish to undergo any operation that could even have the remote chance of interfering with the function of his or her fingers
- If patients have capacity they are permitted to be, in your judgement, irrational
- The job of the doctor is to not only provide information about the risks of the procedure, but also about the benefits that the patient can expect to gain. For example:
  - ' The chance of dying from the heart bypass is about 1 in 100, that is to say 99 in 100 people who have this procedure will leave hospital and hopefully have fewer symptoms'
  - The patient can then weigh this information and make a judgement about whether they would like to proceed
- It can be useful to provide written information so the patient can reflect on what you have told them

FOLLOW-UP

- Ask if the patient has any questions
- Give them time to think about, and weigh up, the information you have given them

CHAPTER 7

Obstetrics and gynaecology

OBSTETRIC HISTORY

INTRODUCTION

- Introduce yourself
- Confirm patient's name
- Confirm reason for meeting
- Adopt appropriate body language

PREGNANCY

General

- Gestation
- Last menstrual period (LMP)
- Estimated due date (by LMP and ultrasound scan)
- Singleton or multiple pregnancy
- Method of conception

Problems

- Hyperemesis
- Vaginal bleeding or discharge
- Abdominal pain
- Constipation, haemorrhoids
- Urinary problems
- Varicose veins
- Movements of baby – should be >10 movements/day in third trimester

Previous pregnancies

- Number of pregnancies
- Delivery – vaginal, instrumental, Caesarean Section
- Sex, weight and development of children

- Complications
  - Intrauterine, neonatal deaths
  - Hypertensive disorders, gestational diabetes
  - Terminations, miscarriages, ectopic
  - Molar pregnancy
  - Preterm delivery

Sexual history

- Pain, bleeding, discomfort during or after intercourse
- Contraception and compliance
- Sexually transmitted infections, unprotected sex

PAST MEDICAL HISTORY

- Last smear test and result
- Endometriosis
- Polycystic ovary syndrome
- Transmissible infections, e.g. hepatitis B, human immunodeficiency virus (HIV)
- Surgical – gynaecological procedures, e.g. LLETZ
- Rubella status (if known)
- Diabetes, endocrine disorders
- Hypertension
- Epilepsy
- Antiphospholipid syndrome/systemic lupus erythematosus
- Psychiatric disorders

BOX 7.1 ANTENATAL SCREENING (SEE SECTION 7, CHAPTER 13)

All mothers in the UK are offered screening for the following:
- Rubella immunity
- HIV
- Hepatitis B
- Syphilis
- Blood group and antibodies
- Haemoglobin electrophoresis for sickle cell/thalassaemia
- Urinalysis (bacteriuria, proteinuria – pre-eclampsia)
- Hypertension
- Down's syndrome and other chromosomal abnormalities
- Spina bifida and other structural fetal anomalies

DRUG HISTORY

- Folic acid supplement
- Iron supplement
- Antiepileptic medications
- Anticoagulation
- Antihypertensives
- Allergies

FAMILY HISTORY

- Diabetes
- Hypertension
- Twin pregnancies
- Ovarian or breast cancer
- Thrombophilia

SOCIAL HISTORY

- Alcohol
- Smoking
- Occupation
- Partner
- Support network

SYSTEMS REVIEW

- All other systems: cardiovascular, respiratory, etc.

OBSTETRIC EXAMINATION

The antenatal obstetric examination, together with history taking during the consultation, is an opportunity to check the health of both mother and baby and to ascertain whether any additional investigations are required.

INTRODUCTION

- Introduce yourself
- Explain the examination and request permission
- Ensure privacy and that a chaperone is present
- Position patient sitting on the couch
- Expose the abdomen

HISTORY

- Ask about the mother's general health
- Enquire about frequency of fetal movement

INSPECTION

- Striae gravidarum
- Linea nigra
- Scars, e.g. Pfannenstiel scar from previous caesarean section
- Rashes
- Oedema (face, hands, ankles, sacrum)

Measure:

- Symphysis–fundal height (SFH) – should equate to 1 cm per week of gestation, and be within 2 cm of this

---

BOX 7.2 DIFFERENTIAL DIAGNOSIS OF ABNORMAL SFH

Small SFH:
- Intrauterine growth restriction (IUGR)
- Oligohydramnios

Large SFH:
- Multiple pregnancy
- Polyhydramnios
- Macrosomia
- Uterine fibroids

PALPATION

- Poles – number
- Lie (after 34 weeks) – longitudinal, oblique, transverse
- Presentation – cephalic, breech using Pawlick grip – finger and thumb
- Engagement – presenting part height above pelvis in fifths:
  - ○ 5/5 – completely above
  - ○ 2/5 or less – engaged
  - ○ 1/5 – one finger breadth remaining above pubis
  - ○ 0/5 – fully engaged

AUSCULTATION

- Pinard stethoscope (over fetal shoulder) – note 'no hands' technique
- Hand-held Doppler
- **Note:**
  - ○ Rate (should be 110–160 bpm)
  - ○ Rhythm
  - ○ Absence of decelerations

FURTHER TESTS

- Check the blood pressure (to monitor for pregnancy-induced hypertension, pre-eclampsia)
- Urinalysis (if required)
- Reflexes, clonus, and fundoscopy (if concerned about pre-eclampsia)
- Ultrasound scan if any fetal concerns
- Blood tests if necessary (pre-eclampsia tests, group and antibodies)

BOX 7.3 SYMPTOMS AND SIGNS OF PRE-ECLAMPSIA/ECLAMPSIA

Symptoms:
- Headache
- Visual disturbance, aura
- Epigastric pain
- Vomiting
- Oedema: peripheral, cerebral, airway

Signs:
- High blood pressure
- Proteinuria
- Hyperreflexia
- Abnormal platelet count, liver function, clotting
- IUGR
- Seizures (eclampsia)

GYNAECOLOGICAL HISTORY

INTRODUCTION

- Introduce yourself
- Confirm patient's name
- Confirm reason for meeting
- Adopt appropriate body language

PRESENTING COMPLAINT

- Nature of any vaginal blood loss
  - Heavy periods
  - Intermenstrual, post-coital, post menopausal bleeding
  - Regular or irregular
  - Quantity – e.g. number of towel or tampons, flooding
  - Quality – colour (fresh or old blood), clots
- Associated vaginal discharge (colour, odour, itching, amount)
- Urinary symptoms: incontinence, dysuria, haematuria
- Abdominal or pelvic pain
- Masses, swellings – especially on opening bowels (e.g. prolapse)

Menses

- LMP; first day of last bleed
- Age of menarche and menopause
- Duration and length of cycle

Pregnancies

- Number of pregnancies
- Miscarriages or terminations/ectopics
- Abnormal pregnancies (e.g. ectopic), labours or deliveries, including instrumentation (e.g. forceps), perineal trauma

HISTORY

Sexual history

- Pain, bleeding, discomfort during or after intercourse
- Contraception and compliance
- Sexually transmitted infections, previous or current
- Last unprotected intercourse

BOX 7.4 COMMON MENSTRUAL PROBLEMS (SEE SECTION 7, CHAPTER 7)

- Menorrhagia – heavy periods
- Dysmenorrhoea – painful periods
- Amenorrhoea – absent periods
- Intermenstrual bleeding

Past medical history

- Last smear test and result
- Endometriosis

- Polycystic ovary syndrome
- Surgical – gynaecological procedures
- Breast cancer

Drug history
- Contraception
- Hormone replacement therapy
- Tamoxifen
- Allergies

Family history
- Gynaecological cancers
- Menstrual abnormalities

Social history
- Alcohol
- Smoking
- Partner(s) symptoms
- Occupation
- Symptoms effect on work/home life

SYSTEMS REVIEW
- Weight change, appetite
- Excessive hair growth, acne
- Change in bowel habit
- Brief questions on other systems: cardiovascular, respiratory, etc.

GYNAECOLOGICAL EXAMINATION

INTRODUCTION
- Introduce yourself
- Explain the examination and request permission
- Ensure privacy and that a chaperone is present
- Ask about painful areas or lumps the patient may have felt
- Position patient lying flat
- Expose from the waist down, using a sheet to maintain dignity

ABDOMEN
Inspection
- Size and shape
- Swellings
- Scars

Palpate
As for abdominal examination – see page 58.

- Begin palpation away from any painful area
- Watch the patient's face during the examination for signs of discomfort.
- Palpate lightly then deeper, over the four quadrants (right and left upper, right and left lower) for:
  - Guarding, tenderness
  - Organomegaly
  - Uterine fundus (quantify size in relation to pregnant uterus)

BOX 7.5 DIFFERENTIAL DIAGNOSIS OF VAGINAL BLEEDING

- Traumatic – e.g. intercourse
- Inflammatory – e.g. cervicitis, endometritis, ulcers, atrophic vaginitis
- Endocrine – e.g. menses, effect of hormonal contraception
- Pregnancy – e.g. miscarriage, placental abruption
- Neoplastic – e.g. endometrial cancer, cervical cancer, benign polyps

---

PELVIS

Position the patient with knees bent and feet together, asking her to relax her knees outwards as far as they will comfortably fall.

Inspection

- Vulva:
  - Visible bleeding or discharge
  - Warts, sores, skin tags
  - Ulceration or lichen sclerosus
  - Visible prolapse

Palpation

- Bimanual palpation (left hand on lower abdomen, right hand per vagina):
  - Size, position and mobility of uterus
  - Cervical excitation (painful cervix on mobilization)
  - Adnexal masses and tenderness
  - Vaginal wall support, uterine or other prolapse

Speculum examination

(See p. 260 for procedure.)

- Cervix and vaginal walls:
  - Cervical ectropion
  - Cervicitis
  - Contact bleeding
  - Cancer
  - Vaginal atrophy with bleeding
- Cervical os:
  - Ulceration or lichen sclerosus
  - Polyps

- ○   Shape – nulliparous (circular), multiparous (elongated, oval)
- ○   Open/closed (in context of miscarriage)
- ○   Bleeding or discharge
- Perform a smear test if indicated
- Take triple swabs if indicated:
  - ○   Endocervical/urethral (for gonorrhoea)
  - ○   Endocervical (for chlamydia)
  - ○   High vaginal swab (for other pathogens)

FURTHER TESTS

- Blood tests: full blood count, urea and electrolytes, liver function tests, glucose, iron studies, clotting screen, LH FSH
- Urinalysis (including β-human chorionic gonadotrophin [LH, FSH, βhCG])
- Abdominal/pelvic ultrasound scan

SPECULUM EXAMINATION

INTRODUCTION

- Explain the procedure
- Gain informed consent
- Explain which tests will be done and how

INDICATIONS

- Abnormal vaginal bleeding: post-coital, intermenstrual, post-menopausal, pregnancy
- Discharge, infection
- Pain, dyspareunia
- Prolapse
- Screening – i.e. cervical smear

CONTRAINDICATIONS

- Patient refusal
- Virgo intacta

PREPARATION

- Obtain:
  - ○   Cusco's speculum
  - ○   Lubricating jelly
  - ○   Swabs (they differ according to site: see Box 7.6)
  - ○   Smear sampling equipment – e.g. Ayre's spatula, cervical brush and glass slide (or specimen pot for liquid-based cytology)
- Arrange a chaperone
- Offer to lock the door of the consulting room
- Ensure adequate lighting

BOX 7.6 VAGINAL TRIPLE SWABS

- Endocervical/urethral – for gonorrhoea
- Endocervical – for chlamydia
- High vaginal swab – for other pathogens

POSITIONING

- Ask the patient to remove all clothes from the waist down
- Ask the patient to:
  - Lie on the couch and cover with a sheet
  - Draw up her knees and with her ankles together, allow her knees to fall open

LANDMARKS AND PROCEDURE

- Warm the speculum under the hot tap
- Don gloves
- Separate the labia with your left hand
- Expose the introitus
- With the blades closed and lubricated, insert the speculum in the lateral position (with handle at 3 or 9 o'clock position), with your right hand
- When fully inserted, turn it through 90° and open the blades. The cervix should come into view between the blades. If the cervix cannot be seen, consider performing a vaginal examination to locate the cervix
- Secure the self-retaining screw on the speculum and maintain downwards pressure to ensure a good view of the vagina and cervix
- Observe the cervical os for:
  - Shape – nulliparous (circular), multiparous (elongated, oval)
  - Open/closed (in context of miscarriage)
  - Bleeding or discharge
  - Contact bleeding
  - Ulceration or lichen sclerosus
  - Cervical ectropion
  - Polyps
- Take appropriate swabs/smear
- Gently remove speculum when finished. Do not close the blades of the speculum on the cervix as this is very painful.

FOLLOW-UP

- Cover patient and allow to dress in private
- Record your findings in the patient's notes
- Label and package any samples appropriately
- Inform the patient when results will be available
- Warn the patient she may experience some light bleeding for 24–48 hours

CERVICAL SMEARS

All women between the age of 25 and 64 are recommended to have a cervical smear every 3–5 years if they have ever been sexually active. This nationwide screening programme aims to identify the precancerous cells of cervical cancer. It does not aim to detect cervical cancer itself.

BOX 7.7 CERVICAL SCREENING

Age (years)	Frequency of screening
25	First smear
25–49	3 yearly
50–64	5 yearly
65+	Only screen those who have not been screened since age 50 or have had recent abnormal tests

source: www.cancerscreening.nhs.uk/cervical

INTRODUCTION
- Explain the procedure
- Gain informed consent
- Explain when the results will be obtained
- Confirm the patient is mid-cycle, do not perform a smear during a period

PREPARATION
- Obtain:
  - Slide labelled with correct patient details (in pencil) or specimen pot for liquid-based cytology
  - Form and bag for sample to be sent in
  - Fixative
  - Cusco's speculum
  - Ayre's spatula or sampling brush
- Arrange a chaperone
- Offer to lock the door of the consulting room

POSITIONING
- Ask the patient to remove all clothes from the waist down
- Ask her to:
  - Lie on the couch and cover with a sheet
  - Draw up her knees and with her ankles together, allow her knees to fall open

PROCEDURE
- Insert speculum and hold firm with your left hand
- With your right hand gently insert the pointed end of a spatula (or brush) into the os and turn it through 360°, and return in the other direction

- Apply a thin film to the slide (or deposit tip into specimen pot for liquid-based cytology)
- Spray with fixative and confirm the patient details on the specimen label
- Remove the speculum

FOLLOW-UP

- Fill in the accompanying form in full including LMP and hormonal contraceptive use
- Inform the patient she may experience light bleeding for the next 24–48 hours
- Confirm when the results will be available and what they may show (see Box 7.8)

BOX 7.8 INTERPRETING SMEAR RESULTS

Potential smear results include:
- Normal epithelial cells present
- Inadequate cells – a repeat smear is required
- Borderline changes – repeat smear within 6 months
- Dyskaryosis

Dyskaryosis indicates potentially precancerous cells – cervical intraepithelial neoplasia (CIN).

The degree of dyskaryosis may roughly correlate with the degree of CIN on colposcopy, but not always – for example mild dyskaryosis on a smear may represent high-grade CIN at colposcopy
- Mild dyskaryosis – CIN 1
- Moderate dyskaryosis – CIN 2
- Severe dyskaryosis – CIN 3

If dyskaryosis is found further investigation may be warranted, according to its severity:
- A repeat smear (e.g. if mild)
- Referral to a gynaecologist for colposcopy (examination and biopsy of the cervix using a microscope), e.g. if moderate or severe dyskaryosis is found

---

PROBLEM PERIODS

Menstrual problems are the most common reason for referral to gynaecology clinics and a common history taking station.

MENORRHAGIA

(Heavy periods, also related to polymenorrhoea – prolonged/frequent periods.)

- Commonly a result of fibroids or endometrial polyps (i.e. increased bulk of the uterus, endometrial thickness and surface area)
- Associated with use of copper coils
- Usually cause microcytic anaemia (iron deficiency)

History

- Women may experience heavy flow known as flooding, and may be afraid to leave the house while menstruating
- Enquire about number of pads or tampons used, frequency of changing

Investigate

- Investigate with full blood count, thyroid function tests
- Pelvic ultrasound scan
- May require hysteroscopy ± endometrial biopsy

Treatment

(Depends on cause.)

- Medical
  - Tranexamic acid
  - Combined oral contraceptive
  - Progesterones (acutely, to stop bleeding)
  - Mirena intrauterine system (IUS)
- Radiological
  - Fibroid embolization
- Surgical
  - Hysteroscopic polypectomy
  - Transcervical resection of fibroids
  - Myomectomy
  - Hysterectomy

DYSMENORRHOEA

(Painful periods.)

Causes

- Normal – common at start of menstruation
- Endometriosis
- Pelvic inflammatory disease (PID) and adhesions
- Ovarian cysts
- Adenomyosis

Investigate

- Pelvic ultrasound in the first instance
- Diagnostic laparoscopy and then:
  - Diathermy of endometriosis
  - Drainage of cysts
  - Division of adhesions

AMENORRHOEA

(Absent periods, related to **oligomenorrhoea** – infrequent periods.)

Causes

- Primary or secondary
- Usually hormonal, but may be anatomical if primary
- PCOS
- Pituitary tumours
- Hypothalmic
- Menopause
- Pregnancy

Investigations

- Full hormone profile (follicle-stimulating hormone (FSH), luteinizing hormone (LH), oestradiol, androgens, sex hormone binding globulin, prolactin, and thyroid function tests, cortisol, 17-OH progesterone)
- Pelvic ultrasound scan

Treatment depends on cause

INTERMENSTRUAL BLEEDING

(Blood loss between periods.)

Causes

- Cervical or endometrial polyps
- Genital tract infections
- Cervical cancer
- Progesterone contraceptives

Examine

- The cervix
- Take genital swabs
- Perform a smear (if indicated)

Treatment

- Conservative: erratic bleeding caused by progesterones will usually settle after 3–6 months of use
- Remove any polyps
- Consider hysteroscopy and endometrial biopsy
- Treat any underlying infection (often sexually transmitted)

MENOPAUSE AND HORMONE REPLACEMENT THERAPY

The average age for the menopause (end of menstruation) is 52 years in the UK although it can occur prior to this (see Box 7.9).

The climacteric (the time to arriving at the menopause) can last from weeks to years. Half of all women will seek help, advice and treatment for their symptoms.

> **BOX 7.9 CAUSES OF PREMATURE MENOPAUSE (OCCURRING BEFORE 45 YEARS)**
>
> - Idiopathic
> - Surgical – e.g. bilateral oophorectomy, hysterectomy
> - Treatments – e.g. radiotherapy, chemotherapy
> - Medical conditions – e.g. Turner's syndrome, hypothyroidism, Down's syndrome
> - Acquired conditions – e.g. mumps, tuberculosis
> - Autoimmune – anti-ovarian antibodies

HISTORY

- Asymptomatic
- Reduced frequency, irregularity or cessation of menses
- Hot flushes
- Mood swings, depression
- Disturbed sleep, lethargy
- Night sweats
- General aches, pains
- Loss of libido
- Vulval dryness
- Dry skin and hair
- Osteoporosis, increased risk of fractures

These symptoms can last up to 5 years, although may be longer.

INVESTIGATIONS

- Diagnosis of menopause is predominantly due to its symptoms and signs
- Measurement of increased FSH levels may aid diagnosis

MANAGEMENT

Complementary therapies

- There are a wide range available in pharmacies and health food shops
- There is limited evidence as to their efficacy and they are generally *not* recommended by professionals for menopausal symptoms

Hormonal treatments

Hormone replacement therapy (HRT):

- Mainstay of menopause treatment
- Provides symptomatic relief but decision to start must be individualized and benefits balanced against the long-term risks
- Protects against osteoporosis and large bowel cancer
- Increases the risk of:
  - Breast cancer
  - Venous thromboembolism
  - Endometrial cancer (unopposed oestrogens in women with a uterus)
- May increase the risk of:

○   Heart disease
○   Stroke
● Contains oestrogen ± progesterone

BOX 7.10 TYPES OF HRT

● Oestrogen only – only recommended for women who have had a hysterectomy/oophorectomy
● Combined continuous – recommended for post-menopausal women
● Cyclical – recommended for women still experiencing periods

---

Tibolone:

● Steroid medication
● Relieves the symptoms of menopause
● Similar risks to HRT

Osteoporosis

● Loss of oestrogens place menopausal women at high risk of osteoporosis.
● Lifestyle changes and treatment options include:
  ○   Avoiding smoking and excess alcohol consumption
  ○   Regular weight-bearing exercise
  ○   Calcium and vitamin D supplementation
  ○   Bisphosphonates (for high-risk patients)

Others

● Some antidepressants may be effective in treating hot flushes
● Clonidine can also be used to treat flushes and night sweats

MISCARRIAGE

First trimester miscarriage occurs in approximately a quarter of all conceptions.

HISTORY

● Asymptomatic (diagnosed at scan)
● Vaginal bleeding (ranging from spotting to uncontrolled bleeding with large clots)
● Previous miscarriage – three or more warrants investigation in a recurrent miscarriage clinic
● LMP and details of menstrual cycle (for gestational age)

EXAMINATION

● Abdomen: soft or tender (should *not* be peritonitic)
● Uterus may be palpable (corresponding to weeks of gestation)
● Observations – per vagina:
  ○   Bleeding
  ○   Cervical os open or closed

- ○ May see or palpate products of conception (POC) within cervical canal (removal with sponge forceps will relieve pain)
- ○ Generalized tenderness (if any) – should not be unilateral

INVESTIGATIONS

- Full blood count
- Group and save
- β-hCG (normally doubles every 48 hours)
- Progesterone level – usually <15 ng/mL
- Ultrasound scan (transvaginal)

BOX 7.11 TYPES OF MISCARRIAGE

- Threatened miscarriage – light bleeding ± pain, os closed
- Inevitable miscarriage – light or heavy bleeding and pain, os open
- Incomplete miscarriage – history of miscarriage or some POC seen, os usually open, retained POC on scan
- Complete miscarriage – history of pain and bleeding and having passed POC, symptoms resolving, empty uterus on scan
- Septic miscarriage – complication of incomplete miscarriage, retained POC become infected
- Missed miscarriage – ultrasound diagnosis, non-viable pregnancy in the absence of pain or bleeding. Gestational sac >20 mm with no fetal pole, or fetal pole >5 mm with no fetal heart movement

---

MANAGEMENT

Most miscarriages will complete spontaneously given enough time – this may not be safe, or acceptable to some patients (e.g. significant blood loss).

Conservative

- ○ Avoids surgical procedure and its risks (plus those of anaesthesia)
- ○ Appropriate for incomplete miscarriage with retained POC <50 mm on scan
- ○ Not very effective for management of missed miscarriage (prolonged)

Medical

- Misoprostol ± mifepristone
- Reduces requirement for surgery by 50 per cent but associated with greater need for analgesia and more vaginal bleeding
- Suitable for incomplete or missed miscarriages in women who want to avoid surgery

Surgical

Evacuation of retained products of conception:

- Quickest resolution of symptoms, most suitable if bleeding heavy
- Most commonly performed with a suction curette
- Risk of uterine perforation, infection, incomplete emptying
- Potential anaesthetic complications

- Most common management for missed miscarriage and incomplete miscarriage not responding to misoprostol

Plus

- Anti-D immunoglobulin should be given to all rhesus D-negative women with miscarriage after 12/40, and women with miscarriage before 12/40 who are managed surgically
- Social support should be offered. Although a common occurrence in hospitals, miscarriage can be very distressing for the woman and her partner

---

BOX 7.12 RECURRENT MISCARRIAGE – THREE OR MORE CONSECUTIVE MISCARRIAGES

Incidence <1 per cent of women of reproductive age
- Uterine anomalies – septum, fibroids, synechiae
- Genetic disorders – sporadic mutations occurring consecutively by chance probably explains many recurrent miscarriages
- Endocrine disorders – polycystic ovarian syndrome, inadequate luteal phase
- Immunological – antiphospholipid syndrome

ECTOPIC PREGNANCY

HISTORY

Features include:

- Abdominal pain
- Presence (or absence) of vaginal bleeding
- Dyspareunia
- Referred pain (ruptured ectopic pregnancy may cause shoulder tip pain)

Gynaecological history
- LMP and menstrual cycle – regular cycle? Reliable dates?
- Gravidity and parity
- Dyspareunia
- Risk factors for ectopic:
    - Increasing age
    - Smoking
    - History of PID/sexually transmitted diseases
    - Tubal surgery
    - Intrauterine coil *in situ*
    - Previous ectopic pregnancy
    - Use of fertility medications, e.g. clomifene

EXAMINATION
Inspection
- Pallor, anaemia
- Lying still or in visible pain

Palpation

- Localized tenderness or peritonism: usually unilateral but may be across the lower abdomen

Pelvis

- Speculum examination – cervical os closed, usually only light spotting or no vaginal bleeding
- Bimanual palpation
  - Cervical excitation
  - Adnexal tenderness (should be unilateral but often tender throughout, especially in presence of free fluid in the pelvis)
  - Adnexal mass or bogginess (free fluid)

OBSERVATIONS

- Monitor for signs of cardiovascular collapse and shock

INVESTIGATIONS

- Urinary pregnancy test
- Serum β-hCG and progesterone level
- Full blood count
- Group and save (if suspect ruptured ectopic cross-match 4 units of blood)
- Urgent pelvic ultrasound scan

BOX 7.13 DIAGNOSING ECTOPIC PREGNANCY

- Pelvic ultrasound scan is diagnostic (in early pregnancy assessment unit if available)

If *ruptured* ectopic suspected and the patient has cardiovascular compromise then patient should go directly to theatre, i.e. this is a clinical diagnosis

Scan findings may show:
  - Empty uterus
  - Ectopic pregnancy, seen directly
  - Free fluid in pouch of Douglas

MANAGEMENT

- Conservative/expectant:
  - Anticipates self-termination of ectopic pregnancy
  - Favoured in asymptomatic patients with a (declining) β-hCG <1000 mIU/mL
  - Intravenous access, baseline blood tests and group and save are still required
- Medical:
  - May prevent the need for surgery and tubal damage
  - Involves intramuscular methotrexate injection
  - Contraindicated if fetal cardiac activity is present (laparoscopy required)
- Surgical:
  - Laparoscopic salpingectomy (gold standard)
  - Laparotomy if patient haemodynamically unstable

Non-sensitized rhesus D-negative women should receive anti-D antibody.

FOLLOW-UP AND COUNSELLING

All cases of ectopic pregnancy should be seen for follow-up in a gynaecology clinic at 6 weeks for review, debriefing and review of histopathology.

INFERTILITY

Infertility is the inability of a couple, having regular unprotected intercourse, to conceive.

- Primary infertility is defined as never conceiving
- Secondary infertility is defined as failure to conceive after having a previous successful pregnancy

It is relatively common in the UK, affecting 15 per cent of couples at some time, with 5 per cent not falling pregnant after 2 years. It is at this point that further investigation is warranted, or sooner if there are related medical problems or the woman is over 35.

BOX 7.14 CAUSES OF INFERTILITY

Men:
- Testicular failure (affects quality and production of sperm)
  - Previous trauma or surgery
  - Infection, e.g. mumps, sexually transmitted infections
  - Testicular cancer
- Semen failure – may be abnormal in number, motility or shape
  - Idiopathic
  - Drugs, e.g. chemotherapy, steroids, disease modifying antirheumatic drugs

Women:
- Age (fertility declines significantly in mid thirties)
- Uterine/fallopian tube failure:
  - Uterine fibroids
  - Endometriosis
  - STIs, e.g. chlamydia
  - Previous surgery, e.g. cervical
- Ovulation failure:
  - Polycystic ovary syndrome (PCOS)
  - Thyroid disease
  - Premature ovarian failure
  - Chemo or radiotherapy
  - Hyperprolactinaemia

Both:
- Stress
- Smoking
- Obesity
- STIs
- Unexplained – 5–10 per cent

HISTORY

- Full medical history including:
  - Past medical history
  - Drug history, e.g. of steroids in men, non-steroidal anti-inflammatory drugs in women
  - Surgical history – e.g. of pelvic surgery
  - Family history – e.g. polycystic ovary syndrome, inherited diseases
  - Obstetric/gynaecological history – including previous pregnancies (see p. 253), contraception, pattern of menses
  - Sexual history – for any previous sexually transmitted infections (see p. 289)
  - Social history – including smoking, alcohol, diet and occupation
- Sexual history – to assess appropriate sexual practice for conception
- Contraception – what and when it was stopped
- Length of time attempting to conceive – 95 per cent take up to 2 years

EXAMINATION

- Gynaecological examination (see p. 258)
- Male genital examination (see p. 293)

INVESTIGATIONS

Men

- Semen analysis
- Sexually transmitted infections – microscopy and culture

Women

- Thyroid function tests
- Progesterone blood test (assesses ovulation)
- Serum prolactin, LH, FSH
- Sexually transmitted infections – microscopy and culture
- Pelvic ultrasound scan, e.g. will diagnose fibroids, ovarian cysts
- Hysterosalpingogram – radio-opaque dye used to assess patency of tubes
- Laparoscopy (and dye) – examines for evidence of structural abnormalities, endometriosis, tubal patency

TREATMENT

Fertility treatment is very expensive and only available free on the National Health Service (NHS) in certain areas of the UK.

Possible therapies include:

- Medication – e.g. clomifene (stimulates ovulation), gonadotrophin supplementation
- Surgery – e.g. fallopian tube or epididymal repair, adhesiolysis, drainage of endometriomas
- Assisted conception – e.g. *in vitro* fertilization, in uterine insemination
- Donation – e.g. of sperm or ova

CONTRACEPTION

There are various methods of contraception that provide varying degrees of protection against pregnancy.

The majority of contraception is available free in the UK to all users.

ABSTINENCE

This is the only failsafe method of contraception.

COITUS INTERRUPTUS

- This ancient method, also known as 'withdrawal', is probably the least effective type of contraception with efficacy rates ranging from 70 to 85 per cent as conception may occur, even without ejaculation.
- It also provides no protection against sexually transmitted infections

NATURAL FAMILY PLANNING

- Colloquially known as the 'rhythm' method
- Involves daily temperature measurement and hormonal urinalysis to calculate the days of the month in which fertilization is unlikely
- It can be up to 99 per cent effective if used correctly but extra contraception must be used during the fertile period of the cycle
- Kits may be costly

DEVICES

Condoms (see p. 295)

- Consist of a thin rubber sheath which is placed over the penis prior to intercourse
- They provide not only protection against unwanted pregnancy but also against sexually transmitted infections
- They can be up to 98 per cent effective if used correctly

Female condom

- They are similar to the male condom
- Inserted in the vagina prior to intercourse
- They are not as effective as male condoms (approximately 95 per cent)

Diaphragm/cap

- These latex devices are inserted into the vagina prior to intercourse to cover the cervix and prevent the sperm reaching the uterus
- They are only 92–96 per cent effective and should be used with a spermicide

Intrauterine contraceptive device (IUD)

- Also known as the 'coil'
- Consists of a small T-shaped plastic and copper device that is inserted into the uterus for up to 5–10 years

- It prevents the passage of sperm and the passage and implantation of any eggs
- This is a very effective method with a failure rate of <1 per cent although is associated with a very slight increase in ectopic pregnancy if conception occurs
- It is easier to introduce in women who have had children

PHARMACOLOGICAL

Intrauterine system (Mirena®)

- IUS is a highly effective form of contraception utilizing the benefits of the coil combined with continuous progesterone release
- Its side effects include those of slight increase in chance of ectopic pregnancy, acne and irregular pv bleeding
- It can remain *in situ* for up to 5 years
- It is up to 99.8 per cent effective

Combined oral contraceptive pill

- This contains oestrogens and progesterone that prevent ovulation and is taken daily for 21 days with a 7-day break each month
- It is 99 per cent effective if used correctly, i.e. correct steps are taken to compensate for any missed pills, vomiting or diarrhoea
- It has several side effects including migraines, weight gain and propensity to hypercoagulability (e.g. thrombosis)– for this reason it is not recommended in smokers

Progesterone-only pill

- As its name suggests this daily pill contains the hormone progesterone
- It prevents conception by thickening cervical mucus (preventing the passage of sperm) and thinning the lining of the uterus, preventing egg implantation
- If used correctly it is 99 per cent effective
- Side effects include acne, weight gain and slight increase in chance of ectopic pregnancy, irregular pv bleeding
- Is safe, however, in older women and those who smoke
- It has a small window of efficacy – i.e. requires a reliable user

Contraceptive implant

- This small, match-stick sized implant is placed under the skin of the upper arm, invisible to the eye
- It continuously releases progesterone for up to 3 years
- It is highly effective with rates of up to 99.5 per cent
- Can be removed at any point and fertility will return very soon after removal
- Side effects are similar to those of the progesterone-only pill

Contraceptive injection

- This intramuscular depot injection of progesterone lasts from 8 to 12 weeks (depending on brand)
- It cannot be 'removed' before that time but provides effective contraception during this period (rates quoted as 97–99 per cent)

- It may take some time for normal fertility to return afterwards
- Typical side effects include weight gain, mood swings, acne, headaches, amenorrhoea and osteoporosis as a result of prolonged use

Contraceptive patch

- This oestrogen/progesterone release patch is alternative to oral or injected pharmacological methods of contraception
- Use and side effect profile is very similar to the contraceptive pill and likewise is up to 99 per cent effective
- A new patch is applied every week for 3 weeks with a 1 week break each month

Morning after pill

- This is not intended as a form of contraception
- Should be restricted for emergency use after contraception failure
- Can be taken at any point up to 72 hours post coitus, although is more effective if taken as soon as possible

SURGERY

Male sterilization (vasectomy)

- This short, simple procedure can be carried out under local anaesthesia
- It involves dividing the vas deferens in the scrotum, preventing sperm from entering the ejaculate
- Claims 99.95 per cent effectiveness (i.e. 1/2000 failure rate)
- Eight weeks post procedure, two semen tests must be negative before use of any additional contraception can be stopped
- Can potentially be reversed later in life, although this can be technically difficult

Female sterilization (tubal ligation)

- This procedure is more invasive and requires a general anaesthetic
- It carries greater risks and a failure rate of 1/200
- It can be performed laparoscopically or via mini-laparotomy
- Both the fallopian tubes are located and ligated (or clipped) to prevent the further passage of any ova to the uterus

ANTENATAL SCREENING

- In the UK all pregnant women are offered routine screening tests to detect the likelihood of fetal abnormalities and infections
- This programme aims to identify fetuses at high risk of genetic or structural abnormalities
- It entails blood tests and ultrasound-based screening
- The initial tests are a safe and non-invasive means of giving parents a quantitative risk of potential fetal abnormality
- This allows the option for further, more invasive prenatal diagnostic tests

BOX 7.15 ANTENATAL SCREENING TESTS

- Rubella immunity
- Human immunodeficiency virus (HIV)
- Hepatitis B
- Syphilis
- Blood group and antibodies
- Sickle cell and thalassaemia
- Urinalysis (bacteriuria, proteinuria – pre-eclampsia)
- Hypertension
- Down's syndrome, other trisomies
- Spina bifida and other structural anomalies

BIOCHEMICAL SCREENING TESTS

- Chemicals produced by the placenta can be isolated in maternal serum
- Abnormal level of these substances, in relation to gestational age, are used to predict anomalies
- This type of screening is most commonly used to predict trisomies and neural tube defects.
- They include α-fetoprotein (αFP), β-hCG, oestradiol (E3), inhibin A and pregnancy-associated plasma protein A (PAPP-A)

Note: Different maternity units have differing screening schedules and tests.

SCREENING TIMETABLE

Booking

- Routine screening blood tests are taken for diseases such as rubella, HIV, hepatitis B, haemoglobinopathy, syphilis (see Box 7.15)

10–14 weeks

Ultrasound scan to:

- Confirm age of the fetus
- Assess nuchal translucency assessment: has a diagnosis rate for Down's syndrome ~80 per cent
- Combined test – nuchal translucency and biochemical screening for trisomies

16 weeks

- Serum screening for pregnancy-related markers
- This may constitute one of:
  - Double test: AFP + β-hCG: 60 per cent detection rate
  - Triple test: AFP + β-hCG + E3 (oestradiol): 70 per cent detection rate
  - Quadruple test = AFP + β-hCG + E3 + Inhibin A: 76 per cent detection rate
- Levels of these serum markers may be influenced by:
  - Maternal weight
  - Insulin-dependent diabetes
  - Smoking
  - Ethnicity
  - Hyperemesis gravidarum

This information must be provided when requesting the above tests and is taken into account, along with the biochemical test results, to assess risk of an abnormal fetus.

18–22 weeks

- Fetal anomaly ultrasound scan is performed
- It can identify structural abnormalities such as cleft palate, cardiac defects or spina bifida
- Decisions about continuing the pregnancy or further invasive screening tests can then be discussed

INVASIVE PRENATAL DIAGNOSIS

Offered to approximately 5 per cent of pregnant women in the UK in whom initial tests produce a greater than 1 in 250 chance of abnormality

Amniocentesis

- Allows fetal karyotyping
- Performed after 15 weeks gestation
- Involves aspiration of amniotic fluid through the abdomen under ultrasound guidance
- Cells are cultured and undergo fluorescent *in situ* hybridization (FISH) or polymerase chain reaction (PCR) analysis
- Results usually take 7–10 days
- Risk of miscarriage associated with the procedure is 1 per cent above controls

Chorionic villus sampling

- Performed from 10 weeks' gestation
- Very early procedures associated with risk of limb defects
- Either transabdominal or transcervical routes
- Aspiration of placental tissue
- Results possible in 48 hours with direct chromosome preparations and rapid cell culture techniques
- Placental mosaicisms can occur in 2 per cent of cases, necessitating further testing
- Risk of miscarriage possibly slightly higher than amniocentesis (1–3 per cent)

MECHANISMS OF LABOUR

ONSET

- Largely initiated by the fetus
- Biochemical factors involved include:
  - Fetal cortisol surge
  - Progesterone decrease, oestradiol increase
  - Prostaglandins
  - Oxytocin

along with changes in tension of the uterine wall

PHASES OF LABOUR

- Latent phase: onset of contractions and cervical ripening. Assessed by Bishop score (see Table 7.1)
- Active phase: regular painful contractions and cervical dilatation of at least 3 cm

Table 7.1 Bishop score:

	0	1	2
Cervical position	Posterior	Mid	Anterior
Cervical length (effacement)	2–3 cm	1 cm	<1 cm
Cervical consistency	Firm	Medium	Soft
Cervical dilatation	Os closed	1–2 cm	3–4 cm
Station	−3	−2	−1 or lower

Total out of 10.

THREE STAGES OF ACTIVE LABOUR

- First – from the start of established labour to full dilatation (10 cm) *should be: 8–12 hours in primiparas, 3–8 hours in multiparas*
- Second – from full dilatation to delivery of the baby *<3 hours in primiparas, <2 hours in multiparas*
- Third – from delivery of the baby to delivery of the placenta *<30 minutes*

FIRST STAGE

Progress in labour is assessed by regular 4-hourly vaginal examinations, to assess cervical dilatation (unless there is an indication to do so sooner)

- Primiparas – 1 cm dilatation/hour
- Multiparas – 1–2 cm dilatation/hour

A partogram is used to plot the progress of dilatation along with:

- The station of the presenting part
- Maternal vital signs
- Fetal heart
- Frequency of contractions

BOX 7.16 THE CARDIOTOCOGRAPH (CTG)

The CTG is a useful tool in assessing the fetal heart rate in conjunction with the frequency and intensity of contractions.

These are assessed by two transducers that are applied to mother's abdomen

A CTG may exhibit:
- A baseline heart rate of 110–160 bpm
- Variability of the heart rate/min (should be >5 bpm) – loss of baseline variability may indicate fetal hypoxia or may be secondary to drugs such as pethidine or methyldopa
- Accelerations of the heart rate – these should occur regularly
- Decelerations – these may be a worrying sign
  - Early decelerations – occur at the start and terminate at the end of a contraction (compression of the fetal head increases vagal tone resulting in bradycardia)
  - Late decelerations – occur after the peak of a contraction and may indicate fetal distress due to hypoxia
  - Variable decelerations – non-uniform decelerations may indicate cord compression or fetal distress

---

SECOND STAGE

Positioning

- Presentation: normally vertex but may be breech, brow or face
- Position: the direction the baby is facing, e.g. occipito-anterior, posterior or transverse
- Lie: this should be longitudinal (cephalic or breech)
- Attitude: this refers to the flexion position the fetus takes up to according to the shape of the uterus, i.e.:
  - Flexion of the neck – e.g. sinciput, face, brow attitude
  - Flexion of the arms, legs – e.g. footling breech, frank breech

Mechanics

- Engagement:
  - This occurs when the greatest bi-parietal diameter passes into the pelvic inlet
  - It may occur several weeks before labour in primiparous patients, or in labour in multiparous patients
- Descent:
  - This gradual process begins with engagement and continues with the aid of the uterine contractions and a thinning cervix, until delivery
- Flexion:
  - This occurs when the head meets the pelvic floor
  - The head flexes, moving from the wider ~12 cm sub-occipito bregmatic diameter to the occipito-frontal diameter (~9.5 cm) to allow passage of the head through the pelvic inlet
- Rotation:
  - The head will normally then rotate from this occipito-transverse position (OT) to the occipto-anterior (OA) position
  - Rotation is completed when the head reaches the ischial spines
- Extension:
  - This occurs when the head reaches the vulva
  - The head crowns when the widest diameter passes through the vulval ring and the head is delivered
- Restitution:
  - The head then returns to its original OT position
  - The anterior shoulder, the posterior shoulder and the rest of the fetus is then delivered

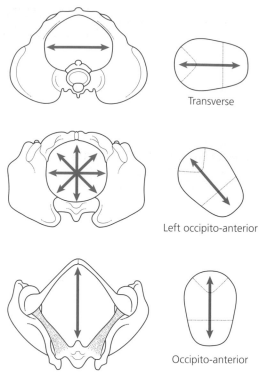

Transverse

Left occipito-anterior

Occipito-anterior

Figure 7.1 Rotation during labour

BOX 7.17 CAUSES OF SLOW/DIFFICULT PROGRESSION OF LABOUR (DYSTOCIA)

'The 3 Ps'

Passages:
- Bony (cephalo-pelvic disproportion, trauma)
- Soft tissue (fibroids, rigid cervix)

Passenger:
- Macrosomia
- Malposition/malpresentation
- Anatomical abnormalities

Power:
- Inadequate contractions

THIRD STAGE

- Physiological separation of the placenta can take anywhere from 5 to 60 minutes
- Active management involves intramuscular oxytocin and ergometrine plus controlled cord traction.
- These hormones promote placental separation and minimize blood loss, which may occur as a result of poor uterine contraction

Paediatrics

PAEDIATRIC BASIC LIFE SUPPORT

An OSCE station testing this knowledge is virtually guaranteed during a paediatric exam and allows you to pick up easy marks, if learnt well.

ALGORITHM

- Check it is: SAFE TO APPROACH
- Is the child: UNRESPONSIVE
- If so: SHOUT FOR HELP
- And: OPEN AIRWAY
  - Head tilt, chin lift
  - Clear any easy-to-remove airway obstruction
- Assess: BREATHING
  - LOOK for chest movement, LISTEN for breath sounds, FEEL for air on your cheek and chest expansion, for 10 seconds.
- Give: 5 RESCUE BREATHS
  - Cover mouth and nose in infant (<1 year)
  - Pinch nose in child and blow into mouth
  - Look for rise and fall of chest wall
- Then: FEEL FOR A PULSE
  - Brachial in infant
  - Carotid in child

Start compressions if no pulse or heart rate <60 beats per minute or unsure.

- Start: CHEST COMPRESSIONS
  - 1 finger breadth above xiphisternum
    - Use only two fingers for infant and one or both hands for child (depending on size)
    - Aim to achieve depression of sternum to one-third the depth of the body
- Ratio of 2 breaths to 15 compressions
  - Rate of 100/min
  - If alone and no help has arrived AFTER 1 MINUTE of resuscitation GO AND GET HELP and in case of an infant, or small child, consider taking them with you

(Source: Resuscitation Council guidelines; http://www.resus.org.uk/pages/pblsalgo.pdf)

FOREIGN BODY AIRWAY OBSTRUCTION

This typically presents a sudden onset of coughing, gagging or stridor and respiratory distress.

Assess severity

- Effective cough – encourage coughing and monitor for deterioration or expectoration of foreign body
- Ineffective cough
    - Conscious – give 5 back blows
        - If no response give 5 thrusts: chest in infant, abdominal in child >1 year
    - Unconscious – give 5 breaths
        - Commence cardiopulmonary resuscitation (CPR)

Back blows

- Infant
    - Place in head down and prone position across rescuer's lap
    - Support head
    - Perform up to 5 sharp blows with the heel of the hand, between the shoulder blades
- Child
    - As for infant in head-down position

Thrusts

- Infant
    - Lie patient supine, across knees, with head supported
    - Locate 1 finger breadth above xiphisternum
    - Perform up to 5 slow chest thrusts, similar to compressions
- Child
    - Sit, stand or kneel behind child
    - Grasp your hands together, one hand holding the other's fist
    - Place hands between the umbilicus and xiphisternum
    - Perform up to 5 short, sharp, inwards and upwards thrusts
    - Avoid contact with and potential trauma to the rib cage

(Source: Resuscitation Council guidelines; http://www.resus.org.uk/pages/pblsalgo.pdf)

NEWBORN EXAMINATION

This screening examination is performed in every neonate prior to discharge.

INTRODUCTION

- Explain the examination to parents
- Request permission

INSPECTION

Top to toe approach

- Skin:
  - Jaundice
  - Anaemia
  - Cyanosis
  - Plethora
- Head:
  - Feel for anterior and posterior fontanelles and suture lines
- Face:
  - Dysmorphic features
- Eyes:
  - Check red reflex (absence suggests congenital cataract)
- Ears:
  - Low set
  - Dysmorphic
- Palate:
  - Important to feel *and* visualize hard and soft palate to rule out a cleft
- Heart:
  - Feel for apex beat
  - Listen for any murmurs
- Chest:
  - Look for signs of respiratory distress
  - Listen for equal air entry bilaterally
- Abdomen:
  - Feel for any masses or organomegaly
  - Check umbilical cord
- Groin:
  - Palpate bilaterally for femoral pulses (diminished in coarctation)
- Genitalia:
  - Check for normal anatomy
  - Ensure both testes have descended
- Hips:
  - Barlow's test – flex hip, push posteriorly – unstable hip dislocates
  - Ortolani's test – abduct hip, pull forward – relocates dislocated hip

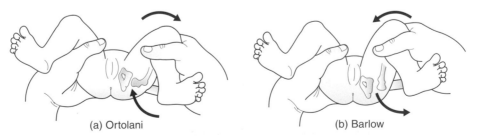

(a) Ortolani   (b) Barlow

Figure 8.1 Hip examination: Ortolani's and Barlow's tests

- Anus:
  - Patency
  - Ask if has passed meconium
- Spine:
  - Check for scoliosis
  - Look for sacral pits or hair suggesting meningomyelocele (spina bifida)
- Limbs:
  - Palmar crease
  - Missing or extra digits
  - Sandal gap
  - Talipes
- Tone:
  - Hypo/hypertonic
  - Normal active movements
- Reflexes:
  - Sucking reflex – infant will suck when something touches the roof of the mouth
  - Moro reflex – startle response to sudden change in infant's position
    - Asymmetry suggests nerve or limb injury, e.g. fractured clavicle, brachial plexus injury
    - Bilateral absence suggests central nervous system (CNS) damage
- Growth:
  - Any lack of subcutaneous fat suggesting intrauterine growth retardation (IUGR)
  - Plot length, weight, head circumference on appropriate growth chart

OTHER TESTS

All newborns are offered:

- Heel prick test: for rare conditions such as sickle cell anaemia and cystic fibrosis
- Hearing screening

POSTNATAL CHECK

All new mothers and babies should undergo a postnatal check-up with their GP or midwife at 6–8 weeks post birth.

BABY

- Complete 'head to toe' examination comprising all systems (see p. 282)
- Weigh the child
- Enquire about:
  - Feeding
  - Growth
  - Gaining weight
  - Responsive and alert
  - Concerns about hearing or eyesight
- Discuss vaccinations
- Complete child health record

MOTHER

History

- General health – eating, sleeping, opening bowels and micturating normally
- Lochia (post-partum vaginal discharge), any residual perineal pain or discomfort
- Pelvic floor exercises
- Breastfeeding
- Contraception
- Keeping smear tests up to date
- Support, coping, psychological issues
- Offer rubella vaccination if antibody negative pre-pregnancy

Examine

- Abdomen
- Blood pressure
- Dipstick urine
- Weigh patient to assess if she has returned to her pre-pregnancy weight

---

BOX 8.1 COMMON MATERNAL POSTNATAL PROBLEMS

- Lack of sleep
- Difficulty opening bowels, faecal incontinence
- Difficulty passing water, incontinence
- Perineal pain and ongoing vaginal bleeding (lochia)
- Dyspareunia
- Breast engorgement, pain, infection
- Poor mood – 'baby blues', postnatal depression

IMMUNIZATIONS

This subject is highly topical and relevant to every paediatric assessment. You may be asked to discuss the risks and benefits of immunization with 'parents' in an OSCE station.

BENEFITS

- Protects against common childhood infections and their potentially life-threatening complications
- Reduces hospitalizations
- Reduces morbidity/mortality, particularly in case of pneumonia and meningitis
- 'Herd immunity' reduces risk to vulnerable patients, e.g. immunocompromised patients
- Reduces socioeconomic burden, e.g. parental days off work

PROBLEMS

- Redness, pain or swelling at injection site
- Febrile illness 1–7 days post administration

- Febrile convulsion 7–10 days post MMR (measles, mumps, rubella) – risk lower than post measles
- Live vaccines, e.g. MMR dangerous in immunocompromised children
- Rarely may induce anaphylaxis

MEASLES, MUMPS AND RUBELLA (MMR) VACCINE

- The Department of Health fully advocates the safety of MMR
- *No* link has been found between MMR and autism or inflammatory bowel disease (as previously claimed)
- There is an inadequate safety profile of single vaccines compared with the MMR
- Reduced uptake of MMR has seen a resurgence of measles outbreaks leading to considerable morbidity and associated hospital admissions
- Measles can have severe sequelae such as:
  - Pneumonia
  - Encephalitis
  - Subacute sclerosing panencephalitis – extremely rare, but devastating and usually fatal
  - Hepatitis
  - Squint
- Mumps can lead to:
  - Deafness
  - Meningitis
  - Encephalitis
  - Orchitis (and potentially reduced fertility)
- Rubella can cause:
  - Serious damage to the fetus when contracted during pregnancy (congenital rubella)
  - Bronchitis
  - Pneumonia
  - Encephalitis

BOX 8.2 UK CHILDHOOD IMMUNIZATION SCHEDULE

Age	Vaccines
2 months	Diphtheria, tetanus, pertussis; polio; *Haemophilus influenzae* type B; pneumococcal
3 months	Diphtheria, tetanus, pertussis; polio; *H. influenzae* type B; meningitis C
4 months	Diphtheria, tetanus, pertussis; polio; *H. influenzae* type B; pneumococcal; meningitis C
12 months	*H. influenzae type B*; meningitis C
13 months	MMR; pneumococcal
3–4 years	Diphtheria, tetanus, pertussis; polio; MMR
12–13 years	Human papilloma virus (girls only)
13–18 years	Diphtheria, tetanus, polio

Source: NHS Immunisation Service (www.immunisation.nhs.uk)

FEBRILE SEIZURES

BACKGROUND

- Febrile seizures are common, affecting 1 in 300 children
- They generally present between 6 months and 6 years
- They are thought to be secondary to an abrupt rise in temperature
- Risk of developing epilepsy is 1 per cent (compared with 0.5 per cent in the general population)

HISTORY

- Typically short, generalized tonic–clonic seizure in conjunction with a febrile illness
- Often positive family history
- A third of children who have a febrile convulsion will have another, but most grow out of it with no future sequelae

---

BOX 8.3 TYPES OF FEBRILE SEIZURES

- Simple – generalized seizure for <15 minutes, no neurological abnormalities or central foci of infection, e.g. meningitis
- Complex – as above but focal, multiple or prolonged seizures
- Symptomatic – as for 'simple' except child has pre-existing neurological abnormality or acute disease

---

MANAGEMENT

- If seizure lasts more than 5 minutes give rectal diazepam or intravenous lorazepam
- If seizure continues, follow advanced paediatric life support guidelines (i.e. phenytoin infusion, rectal paraldehyde)
- Reassure parents (can be very frightening to watch)
- Admit for observation if first febrile convulsion
- Look for focus of infection, e.g. consider lumbar puncture
- **Note:** meningitis and severe bacterial infection can present as febrile seizures
- Prophylactic antiepileptic agents are generally *not* indicated

FOLLOW-UP

- Give parents information on how to manage a seizure, e.g. antipyretics to prevent further occurrences
- Further investigation warranted if:
  - Prolonged seizure (>10 minutes)
  - Focal seizure
  - Focal neurological signs

Genitourinary medicine

SEXUAL HISTORY

Sexual history taking makes many medical students and doctors feel uncomfortable. The key is to practise the questions until they become second nature. It is important to try to overcome these fears by regular practice as a comfortable doctor will put the patient at ease and elicit a far higher quality history.

INTRODUCTION

- Introduce yourself
- Ensure the environment is private and that no one can overhear your conversation
- Use lay language as far as possible – emulate the vocabulary of the patient as far as possible
- Remember the presence of partners, friends or family can often hinder accurate history taking as patients are embarrassed
- Be courteous and non-judgemental
- Reassure the patient that any information disclosed will be strictly confidential

REASON FOR ATTENDANCE

- Ask what is worrying the patient
- Ask relevant questions about the presenting complaint, as per any usual history, i.e. how long has the problem been present, character, associated symptoms
- Go through other common symptoms (see Box 9.1)
- The patient may have no symptoms at all and may want a screen for sexually transmitted infections (STIs). **Note:** chlamydia in particular can be asymptomatic

---

BOX 9.1 SYMPTOMS OF STIS

- Urethral discharge
- Vaginal discharge
- Vaginal bleeding, e.g. post-coital
- Dyspareunia
- Warts

- Rash, itching
- Ulcers, sores
- Abdominal pain
- Testicular pain

SEXUAL ENCOUNTERS

Ask about all sexual encounters in the past 3 months, noting:

- Sex of partners
- Casual or regular (i.e. are they contactable)
- Nature of intercourse (oral, vaginal, anal)
- Insertive or receptive
- Symptoms in the partner
- Contraception

HISTORY

- Significant medical conditions or operations, e.g. Behçet's disease, female circumcision
- Previous STIs
- Vaccination status, e.g. hepatitis B for homosexual men
- For men, ask about urinary or anal problems
- For women, ask about:
  - Last menstrual period
  - Previous pregnancies/terminations
  - Previous smears

DRUG HISTORY

- Intravenous drug use
- Allergies

HUMAN IMMUNODEFICIENCY VIRUS (HIV) TESTS (SEE P. 292)

- Previous test details and results
- Ask about risks for HIV infection, e.g. homosexual men, intercourse while abroad, blood transfusions
- Explain:
  - It is an HIV antibody test *not* an acquired immune deficiency syndrome (AIDS) test
  - About the 3-month window/seroconversion
  - Retesting is required if negative
  - Benefits of knowing, e.g. reduces further transmission, allows planning for pregnancies

DISCUSSION

- Offer to assist in contact tracing
- Confirm confidentiality of records with regards to mortgage, insurance
- Offer advice about safe sexual practice and avoiding STIs
- Ask if they have any questions

POST NEEDLESTICK INJURY/SPLASH COUNSELLING

Sharps or splash accidents are commonplace in healthcare institutions and can be terrifying for the recipient. A calm and methodical approach to a distressed colleague is essential.

INTRODUCTION
- Introduce yourself
- Ensure the environment is private and that no one can overhear your conversation

REASON FOR ATTENDANCE
- Find out details of the exposure:
  - Site of sharps or splash injury (to body)
  - Type of bodily fluid involved
  - Type of sharps involved:
    - Hollow or solid needle
    - Was any fluid injected into the recipient
  - Were gloves worn?
  - Was the site washed/squeezed afterwards?
  - The time of the incident, i.e. how many hours have elapsed
  - How it happened, i.e. the circumstances leading to the accident
- Enquire about the recipient's hepatitis B vaccination status

PATIENT DETAILS
- Ascertain what is known about the source in terms of infectious diseases, e.g. HIV/hepatitis B/hepatitis C
- Are they from an at-risk population, e.g. intravenous drug user
- Arrange patient testing (with consent) for the above viruses
  - (The person who has had the accident should not do this)

ADVICE
- Explain that ongoing care will be managed through the occupational health department (during daytime hours)
- If the incident fulfils the high-risk criteria out of hours, HIV post-exposure prophylaxis (PEP) should be started as soon as possible
  - (Packs are usually kept in the emergency department for this purpose)
- Explain the common side effects of this medication – e.g. nausea, diarrhoea – and that it is thought to reduce the risk of HIV infection after inoculation
- Tell the patient that you will need to take blood from them for HIV, hepatitis B and C and serum store.
- Take consent for an HIV test (see p. 292)
- Advise them to practise safe sex until HIV retesting is carried out in 3 months' time
- Reassure them that even with an HIV-infected patient, the chance of transmission with a non-injected needlestick injury is around 1 in 300 (with triple therapy it is thought to be even lower)
- Suggest that they stop work and go home for the day
- Offer assistance in arranging cover for their shift and informing their manager

CLINICAL GOVERNANCE
- Ensure that a clinical incident form is filled in
- It is good practice to let the line manager/consultant know about the incident so appropriate support and precautions can be considered

QUESTIONS

- Follow-up your consultation by asking if they have any questions

HIV PRE-TEST COUNSELLING

Currently it is legally required to counsel patients when offering an HIV test. This aims to ensure that patients fully understand the implications of the results and make an informed decision whether or not to undergo the test.

INTRODUCTION

- Introduce yourself
- Confirm the patient's details are correct
- Explain what you are going to ask and why
- Be courteous and non-judgemental
- Reassure that the discussion is confidential and that consent is required

PERSONAL INFORMATION

- Sexual orientation
- Ask why they feel at risk

RISK ASSESSMENT (INCLUDE SEXUAL HISTORY, SEE P. 289)

- Sex of partners
- HIV status of partners/contacts
- Condom use
- Nature of unprotected intercourse, i.e. vaginal, oral, anal; receptive or insertive
- Current or previous STI
- Intravenous drug use/needle use, e.g. tattooing
- History of blood transfusion
- Sharps or splash injury (see p. 290)

SYMPTOMS

- Has the patient been unwell or had any symptoms suggesting HIV?
- Possible symptoms of seroconversion include:
  - Rash
  - Fever
  - Lethargy
  - Diarrhoea
  - Sore throat
  - Headache
  - Lymphadenopathy

TEST INFORMATION

- Enquire about previous tests

- Explain
  - The 3-month window/seroconversion period
  - What an antibody test is
  - How testing is done
- That it is an HIV antibody test *not* an AIDS test

RESULTS

- Ask the patient which result they expected
- Ensure they are aware that:
  - They may have a positive result
  - Contact tracing will need to be done if positive
  - They will need retesting if the result is negative
- Inform them of how and when results will be available (usually in person)
- Explain that support is available, i.e. a post-test discussion

BENEFITS OF KNOWING

- Reduces further transmission
- Implications for potential pregnancies
- Implications of taking antiretroviral therapy
- Change sexual practice and risk-taking behaviour, e.g. intravenous drug use cessation and use of support groups

---

BOX 9.2 COMMON ISSUES SURROUNDING HIV

- Uncertainty about the future
- Fear of serious illness and death
- Lack of understanding regarding treatment options
- Change in sexual practice
- Perception from others
- Potential pregnancies and children
- Concerns regarding current and previous partners

DISCUSSION

- Organize a post-test discussion
- Offer to assist in contact tracing
- Reassure about confidentiality of records with regards to mortgages and insurance
- Discuss strategies to avoid risk-taking behaviour in the future
- Ask if they have any questions

MALE SEXUAL HEALTH EXAMINATION

INTRODUCTION

- Explain what the examination entails and why
- Obtain consent
- Offer a chaperone

- Ensure privacy and lock the door
- Ask the patient to remove all his clothes from the waist down

MALE GENITAL EXAMINATION

Inspection

- Look at the different parts of the penis:
    - Shaft
    - Foreskin (if present)
    - Glans
    - Meatus
- Look for anatomical abnormalities, rashes, discharge, ulcers, warts
- Inspect the scrotal sac – remember the left testicle usually hangs slightly lower than the right
- Look for the presence of normal pubic hair
- Look for any lumps in the groins

Palpation

- Penis
- Pull back foreskin if present
- Gently squeeze to try to express any discharge
- Scrotum
- Palpate each testicle in turn gently, feeling for size and consistency
    - Ensure that there are two testes
    - If only one testis is palpable, feel the inguinal canal to see if it can be localized
- Feel for any masses within the scrotum (see p. 293)
- Assess:
    - If you can get above it
    - If it is separate from or attached to the testis
    - For tenderness
- Ask the patient to cough – a transmitted impulse suggests a hernia or a saphena varix
- Transilluminate with a torch
- Feel for masses or tenderness in the epididymis (posterior to the testis) and in the vas deferens

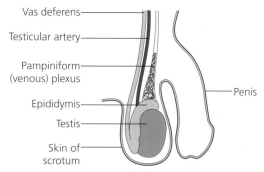

Figure 9.1 Cross-section of a testicle

Completion
- Palpate for lymphadenopathy
- Examine for hernias (see p. 66)
- Go on to examine the abdomen if indicated (see p. 58)
- Cover the patient with a sheet and ask him to put his clothes back on

INVESTIGATIONS
- Swabs, e.g. from meatus for microscopy and culture
- Urinalysis
- Ultrasound of the scrotum to characterize lumps
- Tumour markers (α-fetoprotein and β-human chorionic gonadotrophin (hCG)) if cancer suspected

CORRECT CONDOM USAGE

INTRODUCTION
- Introduce yourself and explain the reason for the consultation
- Ensure privacy
- Ascertain what the patient knows about condoms and their views towards them
- Use lay language as far as possible – emulate the vocabulary of the patient as far as possible
- Explain that condoms prevent against both sexual transmitted infections and pregnancy whereas other forms of contraception (contraceptive pill, coil) are effective against pregnancy only (see p. 273)

INSTRUCTIONS
- Using the condom:
  - Ensure the penis is fully erect
  - Remove the condom from its packaging, taking care not to tear it
  - Roll back the foreskin (if present)
  - Partially unroll the condom to ensure it is the right way around
  - Pinch the tip on the condom and place onto the penis
  - Roll all the way down the shaft
  - If using lubricant, apply to the condom
    - Do not use oil-based lubricants as these can damage the condom and cause them to fail
- Removing the condom:
  - After ejaculation, while the penis is still erect, remove the condom from the penis
  - Inspect for any signs of tearing or leakage
  - Wrap in tissue paper and place in bin
  - Do not reuse condoms
  - Do not flush down the toilet as it may cause blockage
- If the condom breaks:
  - Stop sexual intercourse

- Seek help as soon as possible from a local family planning clinic for advice about emergency contraception
- Remember pregnancy can occur before ejaculation as sperm may be released in the pre-ejaculation fluid

DISCUSSION

- Inform patient that condoms are readily available and free from genitourinary medicine (GUM) and family planning clinics
- Ask if they have any questions

Index

Numbers in **bold** indicate the location of a figure and those in *italics*, a table or box.